How to Die in the Outdoors: 100 Interesting Ways

Introduction

"Man dies when he wants, as he wants, of what he chooses."
—Jean Anouilh, 1960

Anyone can die of heart disease. In the United States, in fact, most people do. The process is time-consuming but simple. All you have to do is eat a lot of fat, give up exercise, smoke (especially cigarettes), drink alcohol heavily, worry and watch the quality of your life fade into oblivion. After a while you'll have squeezing chest pain and shortness of breath before the old ticker, clogged from cholesterol and weak from inactivity, ticks its last and you collapse on the living room floor, the bathroom floor and into your mashed potatoes. How very uninteresting!

In the year 1992, at this writing the last year for which accurate records are available, a total of 2,175,613 deaths were registered in the 50 States, the most ever in one year. These are the Big Ten ways We the People expired between 1979 and 1992:

1. Diseases of the heart.
2. Cancer.
3. Cerebrovascular diseases (stroke).
4. Chronic obstructive pulmonary diseases (emphysema).
5. Accidents (primarily motor vehicle accidents).
6. Pneumonia and influenza.
7. Diabetes mellitus.
8. Human immunodeficiency virus (HIV) infection.
9. Suicide.
10. Homicide.

Basically, if you live a normal boring life like most everybody does, staying indoors most of the time and driving in traffic when you are outside, spending your leisure hours in crowds of people where the sick and the crazies congregate, you have an excellent chance of ending up somewhere on this list. Meanwhile, in the outdoors, close to the natural world of which you are far more a part than you probably realize, there are numerous fascinating pathways to passing on.

This book does not suggest you should quit reading and go out into the wild outdoors seeking death. Life, indeed, is splendidly wonderful and worthy, in most cases, of your keenest attention. If you keep reading, you will actually discover things you can do to avoid ending up dead via the 100 Interesting Ways about which you will soon learn. But, then, when Your Time comes, if you had a choice, it would be a far richer heritage, would it not, to leave behind an intriguing tale.

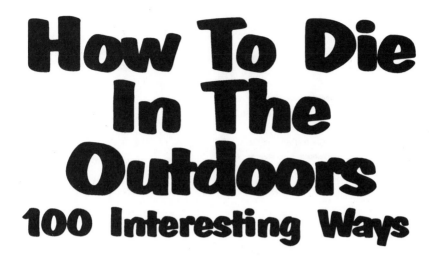

How To Die In The Outdoors
100 Interesting Ways

By Buck Tilton M.S.

Illustrations by Brian Thomas

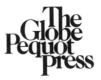

The
Globe
Pequot
Press

Guilford, CT

Previously published by ICS Books.
The text of this book is set in Apollo. Design by Matt Gaylen.

Library of Congress Cataloging-in-publication Data
Tilton, Buck
  How to die in the outdoors / by Buck Tilton.
    p. cm.
  Includes Index.
  ISBN 1-57034-019-6
  1. Outdoor life—Accidents and injuries—Prevention.   I. Title.
  RC88.9.095T54   1995
  613.6—dc20   95-32370

Manufactured in the United States of America
First edition/Eighth printing

Dedication

For Melissa
"It is love, not reason, that is stronger than death."

Thomas Mann, 1924.

And Zachary
"Healthy children will not fear life if their elders have integrity enough to not fear death."

Erik H. Erikson, 1950.

Attacked by Alligator

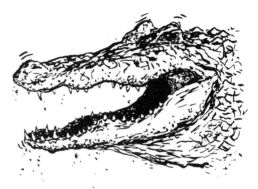

*"Death cancels everything
but truth."*

—Anonymous.

Back when life on earth was young, ancestors of the alligator crawled and swam over the entire United States. They and their relatives (see CRUNCHED BY CROCODILE) have changed little, but the weather changed, people got pushy and now the American alligator (*Alligator mississippiensis*) is relegated to a relatively small area: coastal Virginia to Florida, west to Texas, up the Mississippi River to southern Arkansas. They prefer life wet and mucky in marshes and swamps, muddy rivers and lakes, sometimes the edge of the ocean. They like it hot, but, unlike other crocodilians, the alligator will survive temperatures in the 30s Fahrenheit, although they go dormant in the cold. Mature alligators have reached almost 20 feet in length and over 1,000 pounds in weight.

American alligators can live contentedly for long periods of time between meals. When they are ready to eat, they go out exclusively for a meat dinner, choosing, whenever possible, something bite-size which they can swallow whole, large fish and birds being at the top of the menu. Being unable to chew, the alligator must tear anything too big to swallow into swallowable chunks, an energy-consuming endeavor these reptiles had rather avoid. They rarely take a bite out of humans and, if they do, they are always very upset or very, very hungry. Small adults and children bear the greatest risk for becoming alligator food.

Alligators are experts at attacking. Swimming below the surface of the water, only eyeballs exposed, they silently approach their prey, gambling everything on one swift and merciless attack. If the attackee happens to be you, your first awareness of danger will most likely be the snapping of powerful jaws as they close over a bite-able body part, arm or leg, and the unusual feel of long teeth sinking into your flesh. You will be dragged below the surface and stuffed under a log or into a hole in a muddy bank so the alligator can rip off pieces as the need to eat dictates. Fortunately, you will drown long before you succumb to the pain and horror.

Typically, less than 12 humans are attacked by American alligators every year, and death is not always the result. You could end up in a very small category of Causes of Death.

Moral: *Always swim in alligator-infested waters with someone substantially smaller than you.*

Too High To Handle: Altitude

"What is called a reason for living is also an excellent reason for dying."

Albert Camus, 1942.

Because it's there, you climb a mountain. Each step up in altitude corresponds to a decrease in air pressure. At 18,000 feet the pressure is approximately one-half what it is at sea level. That means every time you suck in a lungful of air you are getting only one-half the amount of oxygen you would get with the same size lungful at sea level. Your body has to adjust to operating with less oxygen, and if it doesn't, you may die of high altitude illness.

Almost everyone who climbs high experiences some of the discomforts of less oxygen: headache, nausea, fatigue, lassitude, loss of appetite, loss of sleep. Some humans go further and start collecting fluid in their lungs, a condition known as high altitude pulmonary edema (HAPE). Why the fluid collects is not exactly known, but it is well known that if enough collects you'll have loss of coordination, chest pain, difficulty breathing and a productive cough. If you don't lose altitude soon enough, you'll drown in water from your own body.

Other humans at altitude, more typical above 18,000 feet, collect fluid in their brain, a condition called high altitude cerebral edema (HACE). A loss of coordination, sudden splitting headache, loss of normal mental acuity and bizarre personality changes precede the point where your brain is squished by the rising pressure inside your head... and you die.

The single most important thing you can do to increase your chances of death at high altitude is ascend as fast as you possibly can. After that, when you start feeling really terrible, stay up instead of going down. Humans who descend almost always recover.

Moral: There's a reason for living down in the valley that only the mountain knows.

The Hug of Death: Anaconda

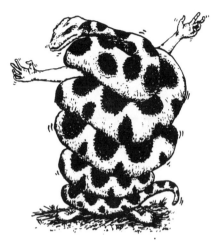

"Is life a boon? If so, it must befall that Death, whene'er he call, must call too soon."
—W. S. Gilbert, 1888.

Of the six giant snakes now living on planet Earth, none grows larger than the anaconda (*Eunectes murinus*), who might surpass 40 feet in length. Living only in the rivers and swamps of South America, the anaconda swims with great agility and speed, a formidable and slim torpedo that could weigh over 400 pounds. Anacondas cannot see well, but they "hear" through their skull bones and "smell" with flicks of their tongues. Their jaws can separate north-south and east-west, ending up attached to the snake only by elastic ligaments.

An anaconda will bite you first with a large mouth full of teeth that curve backwards allowing the snake to hang despite your most vigorous attempts to dislodge it. Terrible but not toxic, the bite becomes the least of your worries as the snake coils its body around yours. Despite myths to the contrary, it is unlikely any of your bones will be broken, a fact that will give you very little comfort. Each time you exhale, and exhale you must, the snake tightens its grip until you are no longer able to draw breath. No breath, no life.

If you are small enough, the anaconda will then unhinge its mouth to a prodigious width and swallow you whole. The digestion process will take a week or more, depending on your size. If you happen to be too big to swallow, lucky you, you will be left dead, useless to the snake. What a waste!

Moral: Never hug anything that eats human flesh.

Annihilated by Army Ants

*"One should die proudly
when it is no longer possible
to live proudly."*
      —Nietzche, 1888.

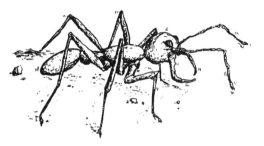

Almost blind, army ants live in colonies averaging 20 to 30 million. Like all ants, they are among the most fascinating creatures of earth, creating social structures among the most complex in the known universe. When the urge strikes, they migrate from one breeding ground to another, following a pheromone trail laid down by the leaders. At an invisible signal, they crowd into a ball while the queen lays her 25,000 or so eggs. Then they march again, and every living thing in their path must flee or perish.

In South America the army ants tend to divide into two columns, forming a pincer movement to trap animals and devour them. Although these ants bite and sting, most humans easily evade the march. In Africa, however, the ants form fronts up to two miles wide and several miles long, pressing on relentlessly unless stopped by fire. Otherwise, they stop at nothing: driving elephants mad, eating horses that were left tied, munching crocodiles caught away from water, even sending anteaters nervously on their way.

They are not fast, moving somewhere between 25 and 50 feet per hour on an average march. But if for some reason you were unable to bolt ahead (downed by a broken leg, staked out by someone who wished you harm), you would be quickly and quietly overrun. Long before you could go insane from the agony, you'd die from the shock of the pain or suffocate as they filled your nose and mouth.

Moral: Those who fear and run away live to run another day.

Abused by Avalanche

"The art of living well and the art of dying well are one."
—Epicurus, Third Century BC.

Any time you have a mass of snow on an inclined surface you can have an avalanche. Avalanches come in two basic types: a loose snow avalanche that releases from one point and fans out as it descends and a slab avalanche that breaks off along a long fracture line and descends, in great tumbling chunks. Both types are typically just waiting for the weight of one human to tip the scales. Snow slides most often on slopes with an inclination of 30 to 45 degrees and, even though avalanches occur on slopes of every orientation, they rumble off north-and-east facing slopes more than south-and-west facing slopes. Broad slopes that curve down into "bowls" and narrow slopes confined by terrain collect the most snow and avalanche the most dangerously. Avalanche danger is greatest during and right after a heavy snowfall and after a period of warm weather, when melting snow consolidates and gets "slippery." One of the primary ways to guess if you're on avalanche terrain is by looking for evidence that an avalanche has occurred there before: rubble at the bottom of a slope, a fracture line at the top of a slope, the absence of trees when nearby slopes are forested, slopes with trees that have their upper side branches ripped off.

Avalanches can kill you in two ways: you are buried and suffocate or you are slammed around by hard blocks until your neck breaks. If you don't want to die, there are several things you can do: (1) When you feel the snow starting to slide, rush horizontally to a safe spot, or at least to a spot where the force of the slide will be less. (2) If you're caught, throw off everything cumbersome and start swimming like mad. (3) Scream once, but after that keep your mouth shut so it doesn't fill with snow. (4) If you're buried, as soon as the sliding snow starts to slow down, start struggling toward the surface, or at least try to clear out a little breathing room for yourself in case someone is looking for you.

Moral: Most death-dealing avalanches are triggered by the human they kill.

Bagged by Barracuda

*"The whole life of instinct serves
the one end of bringing about
death."*
　　–Sigmund Freud, 1920.

More than 20 species of swift, meat-eating fish, family Sphyraenidae, are collectively known as barracudas, but, with few exceptions, they bother humans very little. One exception is the great barracuda, *Sphyraena barracuda*, that grows to eight feet in length, that has a huge mouth filled with noticeably sharp teeth, that has been known to attack humans. Ranging the seas of the world, barracudas bite humans less often than sharks do, but they hit fast and hard, and a five-foot-long specimen could easily remove enough tissue in one chomp to end your life. Loss of blood and the resulting shock would be the cause of your death.

Barracudas couldn't care less about whether or not you taste good. They instinctively bite what might be food. Although ultimately unpredictable, they are stimulated to attack for much the same reasons that sharks bite humans: (1) The water is murky and the barracuda can't tell if you're a regular food source or something new, larger than its normal lunch and possibly unappealing. (2) You are wearing a flashy swimsuit or carrying some sort of shiny paraphernalia that appears to the barracuda to be the belly of another fish or, in other words, a meal. (3) You are an angler or spear-fisher toting a string of bleeding fish, an obvious attraction. (4) You have been messing around with the barracuda, maybe trying to catch it or maybe just swimming in too close for its comfort. And one more thing: big, solitary barracudas are more likely to attack than when they are traveling in schools.

Moral: When school lets out, it's time to go home.

Bombarded by Bee

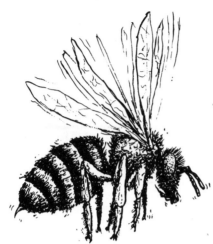

"It is nothing to die; it is frightful not to live."
—Victor Hugo, 1862.

When a honey bee gets riled up, it may deliver a sting to a human with the sharp "needle" in the end of its tail. Each stinger is attached to a venom sac. The venom causes immediate and sometimes frightful pain. When a swarm of honey bees gets riled up and attacks a human, the entire swarm stings at an average rate of four stings per second. If you run away, a wise move, you may have quite a few firey wounds to deal with, but most humans survive just fine. The honey bees do not survive. The stingers are barbed and they rip out of the bee and stay in you, and the bee dies.

Bees, however, and their relatives in the order Hymenoptera (wasps, yellow jackets, hornets, fire ants), kill more humans in the United States every year than all the snakes, spiders and scorpions combined. The reason: anaphylaxis.

Anaphylaxis is a severe allergic reaction brought on by a foreign protein getting into your blood. The protein in Hymenoptera venom causes allergic reactions in many humans. If allergic, you may swell grossly soon after you're stung. But the death-dealing aspect of anaphylaxis, which usually occurs within minutes but can occur hours later, shows itself as extreme difficulty in breathing and in shock. Your face will be red and puffy, and your tongue will stick out as you desperately try to suck air in through your swollen airway. Although you won't know it, your blood pressure will drop dramatically. In a remarkably short time, you'll find yourself losing consciousness. If someone near you doesn't have injectable epinephrine (a bee-sting kit), your spirit will buzz away forever.

Note: Killer bees, slowly migrating north from South America, are slightly smaller and darker than honey bees, but swarm far more aggressively and sting, as a swarm, an average of 24 times per second.

Moral: Bee careful.

Buffaloed by Bison

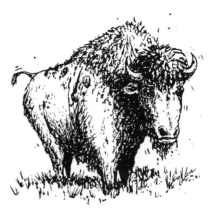

"Let us endeavor so to live that when we come to die even the undertaker will be sorry."
—Mark Twain, 1894.

One of America's greatest losses, bison (*Bison*) once flowed like a vast, hairy sea, numbering in the millions, from the Alleghenies to the Sierra Nevada, from southern Texas to the Great Slave Lake in Canada. Resembling old world buffaloes, North American bison are a different species distinguished by massive, shaggy heads and shoulders and relatively small hindquarters. Unmolested, they are a docile group, what remains of them, not given to harming humans. But when threatened or angered, they have been known to charge.

Often viewed with pet-like affection by tourists to areas where they are protected, bison are sometimes pressed too closely by humans, arousing their sense of preservation. Thundered into by the huge weight and muscle of a bison, you'll go somersaulting, coming to a stop battered, bruised and probably broken. Your day will really fall apart if you happen to disturb an old bull whose herd follows nervously after him. In such a case of trampling, depending on the size of the herd, what is left of you may be difficult to recognize and separate from the chips of dung that typically litter bison feeding ground.

Moral: Don't be a chip off the old bison.

Butchered by Black Bear

"Death is what men want when the anguish of living is more than they can bear."

—Euripides, c. 425 BC.

As far as bears go, black bears (*Ursus americanus*) do not grow very large, maybe six feet and 500 pounds in an extreme case, but they range over a vast area, northern Alaska to Mexico, Florida to California, Maine to Washington State. In color, too, they can range widely: black, cinnamon, blond, blue, brown, almost white. Omnivorous and shy and very strong, they can also be short-tempered. Black bears in many areas have grown quite used to having humans around and, as a result, are turning more and more to humans as a food source. Especially dangerous are older, weaker black bears who can catch and kill little other than a puny, slow-moving man or woman. And to a bear all men and women are puny and slow-moving. As a matter of record, black bears have killed and eaten more humans than have grizzly bears (see GUTTED BY GRIZZLY).

Attracted by thoughts of easy pickings, black bears in recent years have torn through the door of a travel home, climbed onto the roof of a cabin to knock off and eat the human occupant and devoured the arms off of a hiker before leaving her for dead. When you consider the number of black bears and the number of humans, however, bear attacks are still relatively rare.

When black bears do attack a human, there is no intent of playfulness. The bear is hungry. You are food. They seldom bother even to kill you first. They just grab hold and start munching. You may have the exceedingly unusual opportunity to feel yourself being ripped apart and watch the meal, which is you, in progress. Those wishing not to be black bear food report success from attacking the bear back, beating it on the head and face with anything available, including fists, and otherwise resisting consumption as long as strength allows.

Moral: Stand up and fight for your rights.

Beaten by Black Widow

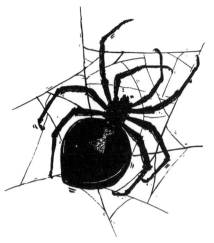

*"As men, we are all equal in
the presence of death."*
*—Publilius Syrus, First
Century BC.*

Wherever you happen to be sitting, or standing or lying, at this moment a spider almost undoubtedly hides no more than a few feet, and certainly no more than a few yards, away. Spiders dominate the non-vertebrate predator world, and, masters of adaptability, live everywhere, from 22,000 feet on Mount Everest to below sea level in the hottest deserts. No less than 36,000 species of spiders are known to exist, divided into over 3,000 genera and 105 families, and, hold on to your video tape of *Arachnophobia*, experts agree at least 36,000 more species wait to be described.

Just about all spiders are venomous. Their poison paralyzes and kills their recently living food, which is usually bigger than the spider. But very few spiders have fangs long enough or venom toxic enough to endanger a human. The black widow (*Latrodectus mactans*) is one notable and dangerous exception, the most potentially lethal spider in the United States.

Female black widows, and only the females can kill you, have been identified in all the Lower 48 States and Hawaii but seem more concentrated in the rural South. Look out for a small, shiny, black, eight-legged creature with a bright mark, typically a red hourglass-shape, on the underside of the largest body part. Being an insect-eater by natural intent, black widows are fond of constructing their webs in insect-abundant places such as below the holes of outhouses. At one time 88 percent of all black widow bites to humans were reportedly to the dangling testicles of males.

Shy and retiring by nature, these spiders do not attack humans on purpose, but are misled by disturbances to their web or caught off-guard by a naked foot stepping on them. Unable to truly bite, they stab and the venom runs down inside their two exquisitely slender, hollow fangs. Although their poison is among the most potent in the world, they carry very little and death to humans is rare, only a few each year, the venom (largely neurotoxic) slowly paralyzing the victim's ability to breathe.

You will usually not feel any pain… at first. If you're having a bad day, 30 to 60 minutes later an excruciating charley-horse-type agony spreads from the bite site to your abdomen, lower back and out your extremities. You may feel weak, sweat heavily, develop a fever, experience a rapid heart rate, drool and vomit. After eight to 12 hours things should start to taper off. However, if you're having a really bad day, your respiratory muscles will gradually weaken to the point where you can't suck air in… and you'll taper off to the point of no return.

Moral: Look before you poop.

Baffled by Bouga Toad

"Death takes away the commonplace of life."
  —Alexander Smith, 1863.

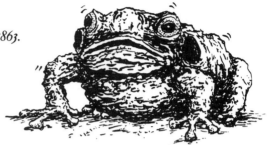

Amphibians (toads, frogs, salamanders) are descended from the first creatures to squirm out of the water and take up residence on land, something that began to happen more than 280 million years ago, and they still occupy that mysterious interzone position: half land animal, half water animal. Of all the groups of vertebrates, amphibians are the most benign to humans. They destroy nothing we want, transmit no known diseases, eat tons of obnoxious insects and have no venomous bites. A few species, however, can cause death to humans in uncommon ways.

The skin of nearly all amphibians secretes some poison, a device they apparently use to protect themselves from something that might eat them (see FINALIZED BY FROG). Some species, notably the bouga toad (genus *Bufo*), a Caribbean resident colored in all the tints of leaf litter, chubby and warty in typical toad fashion, secretes a hallucinogen used by the ancient Mayans, modern Central Americans and Haitian shamans. The toads are against such uses. They get thrown in a pot of boiling water, which forces the juice out of glands behind their eyes. After boiling, the toads are removed dead from the pot. The person who drinks the brew drops over as if dead but resurrects soon to wander around zombie-like doing the bidding of a medicine man or witch doctor until the toad tea wears off. A toad too many, or a swallow too many, and the person who drinks the brew falls over really dead, never ever to rise again.

Moral: Too many toads spoil the broth.

Blasted by Buffalo

"Everything on earth fades fast, Death will take us all at last, that's a truth we know won't pass."

—Georg Buchner, 1836.

True buffaloes should not be confused with American bison (see BUFFALOED BY BISON) and are, beyond a shadow of the bloodiest doubt, the most potentially lethal of all ungulates. In all of Africa the great buffalo (*Syncerus caffer*) is considered by many experts to far surpass the lion and the leopard, the elephant and the rhinoceros, in dangerousness.

Buffaloes are cunning, easily upset and notoriously antagonistic toward any human carrying a firearm especially if they are surprised in dense grass. With heavy, sharp-tipped horns that meet in the middle of their iron-plated skulls, buffaloes have been known to ricochet bullets, dodge hunters and circle around to attack from behind. Their huge bulk is no deterrent to their alarming speed. They aim for a gouge with the horns. Once hooked you'll be thrown into the air, with heights of 10 feet or more common. On the ground, prostrate and bleeding, you have only begun to die. Buffaloes charge back to spear you again. But this time they'll toss their head angrily and mightily from side to side until you have been shredded. So irate is the irate buffalo, one well-documented account reports a human climbed a short tree to escape but could not get his feet above the bull's horns. The buffalo repeatedly slashed the man's feet with its horns until the poor guy bled to death. He was found hanging in the tree, drained of blood. How's that for interesting!

Moral: Keep your guns hidden and your grass mowed.

Bullied by Bull Shark

"You may complete as many generations as you please during your life; none the less will that everlasting death await you."
—Lucretius, First Century BC.

Humans who fish for fun and profit haul an estimated and astounding 100 million sharks over their gunwales every year. These sharks die, often dumped live back into the ocean with their dorsal fins cut off. No wonder some sharks, notably the bull shark (*Carcharhinus*), are apt to take the opportunity now and then to bully a human (see TORN APART BY TIGER SHARK and HAMMERED BY HAMMERHEAD).

Bull sharks probably rip into more humans than great white sharks, and are considered by many experts to be the most dangerous man-eater in tropical seas. One reason bull sharks rate high on the danger list is an unusual habit they have: they swim regularly up into fresh water rivers, including the Amazon (South America), Bombay (Asia), Brisbane (Australia), Congo (Africa) and lower Mississippi (good ole USA). Brown, black or gray in color, growing to 11 feet in length, bull sharks can weigh well over 400 pounds. Among the least picky about their food of all sharks, bulls are wonderfully opportunistic, eating whatever whenever they have a chance, but feeding primarily at dawn and dusk. Beady of eye and blunt of nose, these sharks have a very large mouth filled with very large serrated teeth. If you're a target, they'll raise their snout to perfectly line up their gaping jaws for a bite, which will remove a very large portion of you.

Here are five ways of increasing the odds of a shark attack: (1) Swim with sharks. (2) Bleed while swimming with sharks. (3) Swim in murky water. (4) Swim alone. (5) Swim at night.

Moral: Nobody likes a bully.

Chewed by Camel

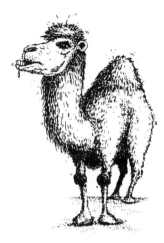

"Death is a camel that lies down at every door."
— *Persian Proverb.*

All the hoofed animals of the world are collectively known as ungulates. They are divided into two orders depending on whether they have an odd number of toes (such as horses, rhinoceroses and tapirs) or an even number of toes (such as pigs, cows, sheep, goats, deer, llamas and camels). Though generally docile, there are notable exceptions (see Blasted by Buffalo). To the exceptions you may add camels.

The Arabian camel, *Camelus dromedarius*, has one hump and is used as a beast of burden in hot, sandy regions such as Arabia and Africa. The Bactrian camel, *Camelus bactrianus*, has two humps and is seen most often in cooler, rockier areas such as Asia.

Camels are known around the world for their ability to store large amounts of water and go for long days and long miles without refreshment. They are less known for but just as liable to be foul of temper and fly off the handle when overloaded. Indeed, overburdened dromedaries will secretly hold intense hatred for an abusive handler, biding their time and attacking when least expected. They attack with their teeth. Camels, unlike most herbivores, have canine teeth which have been known to sever a human's limb. If your limb doesn't sever, they'll lift their heads up and back, flipping you around with enough force to literally break your neck. If that doesn't work and they get you on the ground, they'll keep biting until you bleed to death. One hump or two? Who cares? Your screams will not bother them in the least.

Moral: Don't be a burden to others.

Canned by Candiru

"Death in itself is nothing; but we fear to be we know not what, we know not where."

–John Dryden, 1682.

The size of a small toothpick, an inch or so long, the candiru is an almost invisible catfish, an inhabitant of Amazonian waters, a parasite (which is most unusual among fish). The candiru sucks blood, most often by attaching itself to the gills of larger fish and drinking until it is satiated and dropping off to rest on the bottom until it gets hungry again. To the utter devastation of numerous humans, mentally and sometimes physically, the candiru has a serious problem distinguishing between the smell of blood-rich fish gills and the smell of human urine. They swim up into the urethra of peeing people, or into other urogenital openings. They expand their spikelike gills, which hold them within the gills of other fish while they feed, after which they swim on forward and out. In a human urethra there isn't an out to swim. They are very, very securely stuck inside. Called urethra fish in English (candiru is Brazilian), the minuscule catfish will swim on eventually into your bladder, you get all septicemic ("blood poisoned") and you die.

In Amazonian males, early methods of treatment included whacking off, in a most literal sense, the penis. This may help explain the low population growth rate for Amazonians. Large doses of citric acid have now been proven to soften the spikelike gills and often encourage the release and resulting expulsion of the candiru. In female humans who want to live, this is the only hope.

Moral: The Amazon Basin may be an excellent opportunity for someone who sells snug-fitting swimsuits.

Croaked by Cane Toad

"He hath lived ill that knows not how to die well."
—Thomas Fuller, 1732.

Four to nine inches long and up to four pounds in weight, cane toads are big and fat, greenish-yellow and able to put rabbits to shame with their ability to reproduce. A pair of cane toads would produce 60,000 more toadies every year if all their eggs became mature adults. Hopping rampant in Australia, feeding at night, these amphibians were imported once upon a time from South America so the toads would eat beetles attacking sugar cane fields. Taking a liking to Down Under, the toads proliferated to the point where they're thicker than fleas on a dingo's back. In addition to insects, cane toads will eat meat, including small birds and each other. Crushed, the toads stink vilely, but that's only a small part of the problem.

Two glands on the sides of their wart-strewn bodies constantly secrete a venom called bufotenine. When the cane toad is pressured, the secretion rate will increase, and, when the cane toad is really upset, the venom will shoot out for up to 40 inches, causing temporary blindness if it lands in your eye. Anything attempting to eat a cane toad, a really upsetting experience for the toad, dies from the poison. A growing number of humans with questionable intelligence remove and dry the toad's skin and smoke it for what is reportedly an acceptable high. A growing number of the growing number are dying. On the ragged edge of humanity, a few have actually licked the toad for the hallucinogenic effect. Now there's an interesting way to croak.

Moral: Unlike most humans, toads can take a licking and keep on kicking.

Carved Up by Cannibal

"Life is a great surprise. I do not see why death should not be an even greater one."

—Vladimir Nabokov, 1962.

Nothing in your wildest imaginations has come near to ending as many human lives as other humans: wars, homicides, inquisitions. Over the years a surprising number of those human deaths have been followed by a feast in which the dead human was dinner for fellow humans. After their hearts had been torn out on altars, the Aztecs regularly fed on the bodies of their sacrifices, usually stewed with tomatoes and peppers. The Senga country of Africa has a long history of cannibalism dating back well before the first historians started making notes on African eating habits. Whether or not they threw living missionaries into pots of boiling water remains a moot point, unless you were one of the missionaries. When Columbus "discovered" America, he was warned to stay off several islands of the Indies where the Carib Indians were very fond of roasting and consuming invited and uninvited humans. The word "barbecue," in fact, is a Spanish corruption of the Indian word for their roasting device. Many famous lost-in-the-wilderness incidences have become famous because the survivors ate the dead.

Even more startling is the number of cannibals who still today break their fasts on leg of man or arm of woman. This is mostly done in areas where McDonalds and microwaves do not exist, and mostly done by one primitive tribe to another whose flavor has found favor. If you wandered in at meal time, however, there's no reason to think you might be spared. Fine chefs, it seems, will always butcher you first and add a few condiments, so at least you won't have to wait for the water to boil.

Moral: You never know who's coming for dinner.

Done In by Cape Hunting Dog

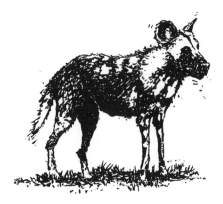

"It hath often been said, that it is not death, but dying, which is terrible."
—Henry Fielding, 1751.

Domestic dogs occasionally show up in the news as killers and, rarely, eaters of owners or, even more often, of neighbors or postal service workers. Dobermans and pit bulls account for many of these accounts, but their attacks are often indoors or, at least, in the backyard, and they really don't qualify, even though they're interesting, as outdoor deaths. But domestic dogs have close relatives in the wild outdoors, true wild dogs, the Canidae, which include the Cape Hunting Dogs (*Lycaon*), the small, big-eared canines of Africa.

Wild dogs travel in groups called packs and are extremely opportunistic feeders: if they get the opportunity, they feed. Being relatively keen of intelligence, Cape Hunting Dogs fear humans and shun them most of the time. A lone human, however, to a hungry pack might well become dinner.

Working as a well-coordinated team, the dog pack will surround you. A rush by one dog can be turned with a kick or a blow to its nose with a stick or rock. But while you're striking at dog one, dog two runs in to tear out one of your leg muscles with sharp teeth powered by crushing strength. Once you're on the ground, it's all over in a matter of seconds: a half-dozen dogs are savaging your arms and legs off while one brute rips out your throat. For what it's worth, in the spirit of the finest environmentalists, none of you will go to waste.

Moral: Let sleeping dogs lie.

Castrated by Cassowary

"Neither the sun nor death can be looked at steadily."
—La Rochefoucauld, 1665.

One of the few, perhaps the only bird to go out of its way to attack humans, distant relatives of the ostrich and emu, the six species of cassowaries (genus *Casaurius*) live only in Australia, New Guinea and adjacent islands. Generally greenish in color, loose and coarse, their plumage hangs down like thick hair that has lost its interest in life. With wings too small for flight, cassowaries reach five feet high at maturity and run speedily across the ground on enormously powerful legs that end in feet with a long, straight, strong, sharp claw on each of the two innermost toes. Since they choose one mate and stick together, when you see a lone cassowary it probably isn't. The other one is lurking nearby.

Remarkably dumb with a reputation for "flying" completely into hysterics, quarrelsome and combative in nature, cassowaries, when surprised in the bush, tend to charge regardless of what disturbed them. Before slamming into you, at a precisely timed moment, they'll leap into the air and slash out and down with their knife-like claws. Any part of you in the path of the claws will be ripped open the way you tear into a resistant bag of corn chips. The attack may be formidable and prolonged, depending on how resistant you are. If you are suddenly overcome with a deep desire to see tomorrow, forget outrunning a cassowary. Try throwing yourself to the ground, curling up and covering everything vital with your arms, and hoping for the best.

Moral: Birds of a feather freak out together.

Censured by Centipede

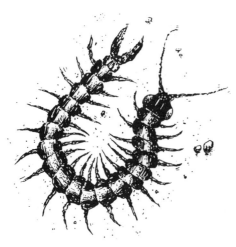

*"Our repugnance to death
increases in proportion to
our consciousness of having
lived in vain."*
—William Hazlitt, 1817.

Centipedes, those creatures of a hundred feet, differ from millipedes, those of a thousand feet, in a couple of ways. For one thing, centipedes, around 1,500 species, have a pair of feet per body segment (not always exactly 100) while millipedes, about 6,500 species, have two per body segment which, by the way, numbers a millipede's feet around 200 and a far piece from a thousand. For another thing, centipedes are carnivores and millipedes are vegetarians. Centipedes grab their prey with claw-like jaws and induce venom from glands at the base of their jaw.

When centipedes bite you it will hurt and that's about it. If it happens, however, to be a *Scolopendra heros* of the southwestern United States, a centipede achieving six to eight inches in length, the pain can be extreme and the venom can cause serious complications, including dizziness, nausea and collapse with possible massive swelling near the bite, loss of motor function and even loss of muscle tissue. Death, so far, appears to not happen.

But in the tropical regions of Asia centipedes grow to a foot in length and regularly eat small birds and mice for a living. Although information on tropical centipedes is scarce, reports indicate Indian and Burmese centipedes have kept human victims bedridden for over three months, Sri Lankan centipedes have caused human deaths, and centipedes from Malaysia have bites worse than some of the local vipers.

*Moral: Never trust anything with more feet than you and your
entire high school biology class combined.*

Sunk by Ciguatera

"In the depth of the anxiety of having to die is the anxiety of being eternally forgotten."

—Paul Tillich, 1963.

More commonly diagnosed than any other fish-related illness, ciguatera poisoning follows ingestion of several types of tropical and subtropical reef fish in the Pacific and Caribbean, especially but not only: snapper, grouper, kingfish, amberjack, barracuda, dolphin (the fish one), wrasse, surgeonfish, goatfish and parrotfish.

Tiny dinoflagellate marine algae called *Gambierdiscus toxicus*, when eaten by herbivorous reef fish, produce toxins that concentrate in the fishes guts. Among those toxins are ciguatoxin and ciguaterin. When humans eat these vegetarian fish, or the carnivorous fish that have eaten the vegetarians, poisoning occurs. What happens in the sea to produce the dinoflagellates is not known. It's a big problem for fish-eaters who want to live in the South Pacific, Japan, the Bahamas, Hawaii, Puerto Rico or Florida, and ciguatera has been diagnosed at least two dozen times in Baja.

Ciguatera toxins give the fish no unusual odor, taste or color, and they are resistant to freezing, cooking, drying and smoking. Within 24 hours of ingestion, you'll usually complain of gastrointestinal symptoms: nausea, vomiting, abdominal pain, diarrhea. In mild poisonings these symptoms resolve quickly, but they may last for as long as a week. Neurologic symptoms include paresthesia (strange skin sensations), vertigo, ataxia (loss of coordination), myalgia (muscle pain), weakness, headache, cold/hot sensory reversal, joint pain and itching. Most weird is an occasional complaint of feeling like your teeth are loose. These symptoms, too, spontaneously resolve, but may reoccur from time to time over the next few years. Cardiovascular symptoms occur only in victims who have been severely poisoned and may include tachycardia (fast heart rate), bradycardia (slow heart rate) and hypotension (low blood pressure). Sometimes symptoms are worse on a second exposure to the toxins. Death is rare but has been reported.

Moral: There's something more than fishy about some fish.

Captured by Giant Clam

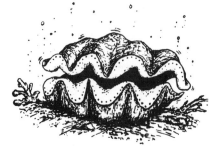

*Every death even the cruellest
Drowns in the total indifference
of Nature
Nature herself would watch
unmoved
If we destroyed the entire
human race.*
                    —Peter Weiss, 1964.

Pearl divers of the Indo-Pacific region, off many South Pacific island groups and off the coast of East Africa insist that the giant clam (*Tridacna gigas*) is a threat to life. Without their shells the soft body parts may weigh in at 20 pounds or more, a hefty meal for the mollusk-eater but hardly a menace. The shell, however, of this humongous bivalve (sometimes called the killer clam or man-eating clam) may exceed four feet in length and 500 pounds in weight. The strength of the adductor muscles required to shut the shell, as you can imagine, is immense.

The *U. S. Navy Diving Manual* rates the giant clam a 2-plus (out of a possible high mark of 4-plus) on the danger scale, and says: "Traps arms and legs between shells." With serrated edges, the two halves of the shell fit together like the jaws of a mighty bear trap and as tight as a pearl-buyer holds onto money.

On behalf of giant clams let it be known they do not eat humans. Victims simply freak out and struggle until they drown. A vast weight of evidence indicates tridacna clams are innocent undersea bystanders prompted by nothing other than a tickle to their "trapdoor."

Moral: Never look a gift pearl-bearer in the mouth.

Clobbered by Cobra

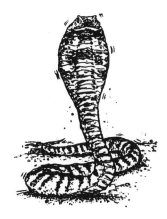

"Death will not see me flinch;
the heart is bold that pain
has made incapable of pain."
     –Dorothy Parker, 1926.

The Elapidae family of snakes (kraits, coral snakes and cobras) includes about 230 species, of which all are venomous. Few snakes on earth, maybe none, have received as much publicity as cobras, inhabitants of Africa and Asia, distinctive partially due to their impressive "hoods" which fan out from their necks via special little rib bones. The famous asp of Egypt, immortalized in so many statues, killer of Cleopatra, is an Egyptian cobra (*Naja haje*). The fascinating snake charmers of India musically entice common cobras (*Naja naja*) sinuously up from baskets. The mighty King cobra (*Ophiophagus hannah*), star of numerous tales, has been measured at almost 19 feet in length and possesses, agree the experts, the deadliest snake bite on earth at least partly due to its great size.

Cobras all possess short, hollow, fixed fangs and neurotoxic venom (which means the venom attacks the central nervous system instead of rushing around in the blood and causing damage the way a hematoxic venom does). Cobras, the King cobra being an exception, generally don't mind living near and biting humans on a regular basis.

Perhaps the most universally feared elapid is the spitting cobra (*Naja nicricollis*), an irascible animal with the nasty habit of literally spitting its venom from holes in the front of its fangs distances up to around seven feet, with great accuracy. It always aims for the eyes, and the venom causes severe pain and blindness long enough for the snake to slither in for a deadly bite. You'll feel pain when it bites, too, and you'll swell near the site of the bite. You'll get weak and drowsy, have trouble seeing and swallowing, develop a headache, lose your ability to talk, drool, throw up, go numb and partially paralyzed, convulse and slip into complete paralysis, including the muscles that power your breathing, so you die.

Moral: There can be more to wearing glasses than just seeing better.

Conked by Cone Shell

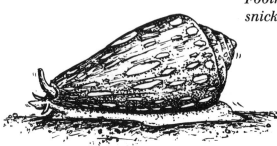

*"I have seen the eternal
Footman hold my coat, and
snicker."*

−T. S. Eliot, 1915.

Among the most delicate and beautiful of color of any seashells, there are between 400 and 500 species of cone shells (genus *Conus*), and they are all equipped with a highly developed apparatus for envenomation. Found in tropical and subtropical seas, cone shells live on rocks and coral and sometimes are seen crawling along sandy bottoms. Generally shy and retiring, the animals inside the shells hide when approached. But they strike out violently when the shell is handled.

Once in your hand, a snout shoots out of the cone shell's opening, a fleshy snout of remarkable length. The snout contains quite a few rigid, hollow tools called radula teeth, which will quickly penetrate your skin, even through gloves. The wound looks like a scrape. Each harpoon-like tooth has its own separate venom supply which enters your body. On the low end of "bad," some cone shell venom provides pain like the worst bee sting you can imagine while on the upper end death has occurred in less than four hours. With a 20 percent mortality rate, cone shells rank statistically higher than cobras and rattlesnakes as death dealing devices.

Besides pain, you should feel tingling and numbness, especially in your lips and mouth, followed shortly by a creeping paralysis in your arms and legs. Be prepared for some dizziness and vomiting. As the paralysis spreads to your diaphragm, you'll find it more and more difficult to first talk and then breathe. If you got scraped by one of the less venomous species, these problems will pass. If you handled one of the more venomous species, you will soon lose consciousness and expire.

Moral: Keep your hands to yourself.

The Kiss of Death: Conenose Bug

"Death is given in a kiss..."
—Robert Louis Stevenson, 1878.

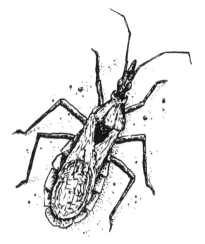

Smooth and oval-shaped, brownish in color, the conenose bug (or kissing bug, or assassin bug) is a *Triatominae*, a *vinchuca* to Spanish-speaking humans (meaning "one who lets himself fall down"). Less than an inch long, conenose bugs have long, narrow cone-shaped heads with two antennae and a proboscis that curves under. On the sides of the abdomen you might see narrow stripes of light yellow or red. It uses its two pairs of wings like a parachute to drop out of bushes and thatched roofs onto the faces of sleeping humans to feed on blood.

Once comfortable, most often near your mouth, the bug "kisses" with a scalpel-like extension of its proboscis and sucks your blood for about 20 minutes, ingesting many times its own weight. As it feeds, it poops, and its poop contains a parasite, *Trypanosoma cruzi*, the cause of Chagas' disease. You rub your irritated wound after the bug leaves, you rub the parasite into you and you get really sick.

This is how it works. After about one week, you'll develop a hard, violet-hued bump where the bug bit. The parasites, clustered at the bump, begin to disperse throughout your body in your bloodstream. They invade your heart, brain, liver and spleen. In children, a severe brain infection may occur and lead to death. In adults, the primary effect is on the heart, where lesions form that gradually reduce the effectiveness of your blood-pumping muscle.

Some humans die in three months or so. Most humans survive initially to slowly succumb to the disease over the next 10 to 20 years. During those years the infected human passes the disease to other human, via the conenose bugs who feed on one human one time and another the next time. Currently an estimated 16 to 18 million Latin Americans are dying from the kiss of death.

Moral: A stolen kiss can steal your life.

Corralled by Coral Snake

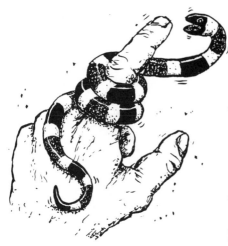

*"The nearest friends can go
with anyone to death comes
so far short they might as
well not try to go at all."*
    —Robert Frost, 1914.

All of the poisonous snakes in
the United States are either members of the family Crotalidae (see
RIPPED BY RATTLESNAKE) or the
family Elapidae which includes, in North America, two genera: *Micrurus*
(the Southeastern, Florida and Texas coral snakes) and *Micruroides* (the
Sonoran coral snake). Among the most brightly colorful animals on the
continent, coral snakes are banded in brilliant red and yellow and shiny
black. They are often confused with the equally colorful and harmless
scarlet king snake, but the order of the colors differs. If red is bordered on
both sides by black, the snake will not harm you. If red is bordered on
both sides by yellow (or sometimes white), the snake is venomous.

Slim and rarely reaching two feet in length, without an enlarged head,
coral snakes are shy and reclusive, with a primitive venom system that
includes two short, fixed, relatively dull fangs in the front of the upper
jaw. They cannot strike out and rip through clothing and, indeed, must
literally chew for several seconds in order to break your skin and shoot
you up with a very potent neurotoxic venom.

If you are silly enough to let a coral snake gnaw its way through your
skin, you probably will feel little or no pain and see no swelling. Within
about 90 minutes, however, you should start to feel weak or numb, especially in the bitten arm or leg. A few hours later you'll start to drool and
shake. You may feel drowsy. Somewhere in the five to 10 hour range after
the bite, you'll find it difficult to talk and then breathe. When you can't
breathe at all, you'll die.

The rare human gets bitten by a coral snake in the United States, and
rarer still the one who dies. If you happen to see a coral snake, and you
rush over and grab it and shake it, and then let it chew on you for a while,
you could be one of a few. You will also be very deserving of your death.

Moral: Red on yellow kills a fellow… or a woman.

Consumed by Cougar

"Death is stronger than all the governments because the governments are men and men die and then death laughs: now you see'em, now you don't."

—Carl Sandburg, 1950.

Mountain lion, puma, panther, catamount or cougar, all the names point to one animal, *Felis concolor*, the largest wild cat of the United States, a feline that might reach a weight of 200 pounds. Once roaming with quiet dignity from southern Canada to the tip of South America, in forest and in field, cougars now are seen rarely outside the wildest areas of the western United States except very rare sightings in the swamps of Georgia and Florida. Still, no cat on earth has adapted to as broad a range of latitudes or habitats as the cougar.

No doubt exists whatsoever that mountain lions would greatly prefer to never see a human being. As their habitats become increasingly cluttered with humans, however, a simultaneous and slight increase in cats viewing humans as food has naturally occurred. Cougars may also attack if cornered, the attack being announced by its ears being laid back, snarls and tail-twitching. As with all cats, cougars may be attracted to you by simple curiosity, become frightened and kill.

Cougars are powerful, with long sharp claws and long sharp teeth. Like most feline predators, they would much rather you not know they were coming in for a kill. A slinking up, a sudden pounce, teeth closing over your neck and you're dragged to the ground perhaps never knowing what broke your neck. The claws, although capable of causing great damage, are primarily used for holding on in case you survive the initial attack and try to get away. If you do survive, and wish to go on living, evidence suggests a strong counter-attack on your part might well scare the cat off. Otherwise the hungry cougar will eat you.

Moral: Curiosity kills more than cats.

Cracked by Crab

"Grieve not; though the journey of life be bitter, and the end unseen, there is no road which does not lead to an end."
—Hafiz, Fourteenth Century AD.

Humans have regularly hunted crabs for food ever since that distant day when someone discovered they tasted good. On the shores and islands of the South Pacific, the Indian Ocean and the adjacent seas, lives a much sought after crustacean, *Birgus latro*, the robber crab or coconut crab, growing to over a foot in length and culinarily just fine when boiled, cracked open, the meat picked out and dipped in warm butter. Crabs have always had a chance to return the compliment when a dead human ended up in their domain, although they simply tear a corpse apart and eat it disgustingly soggy and raw. Coconut crabs get some direct revenge by commonly carrying a toxin that can make humans sick. Occasionally, if truth be told, very rarely, *Birgus* does more.

Called coconut crabs for a remarkable reason, these creatures scuttle sideways from the sea to climb palms and pinch off coconuts, causing them to fall to the sand. Then they descend to tear the coconuts apart with their tremendously powerful pincers. Then they eat the coconut.

At least one account from 1951, from an island in the Red Sea, reports that shipwrecked Moslem sailors were dozing weakly on the beach. Coconut crabs emerged silently from their salty home to crack open the skulls (and kill) 26 humans before the survivors awoke and retaliated. Perhaps the crabs mistook the hairy human heads for coconuts. Perhaps the crabs, at last, had an opportunity for true revenge.

Moral: Bald is beautiful.

Crunched by Crocodile

"It is as natural to die as to be born."

–Francis Bacon, 1625.

True remnants of the Age of Reptiles, the only living descendants of the most successful class of land vertebrates ever, crocodiles and their relatives (see ATTACKED BY ALLIGATOR) have changed little in the last 70 million years or so. One alteration in crocodiles is that they once grew to more than 50 feet in length. Today, if you're lucky… or unlucky… you may see a crocodile (*Crocodylus acutus, Crocodylus intermedius*) reaching 23 feet from snout to end of powerful tail. They like their weather really hot and are found in all tropical regions of the earth: northern South America, southern North America, Africa, India, Southeast Asia, northern Australia and other such places.

No animals on earth, with the possible exception of a few sharks (see GOBBLED BY GREAT WHITE SHARK), are as totally dedicated to eating meat. On a lazy day, when the pickings are slim, crocodiles are well known devourers of their own young.

The smell of blood immediately arouses crocodiles. They will slide silently and efficiently into the water, approaching a bleeding victim with immense strokes of their tails even when they aren't especially hungry. Far more aggressive and voracious than their alligator cousins, crocodiles think nothing of attacking something quite a bit bigger than an alligator would ever even consider attacking. In regions of the world where registration of the dead is not required, crocodiles crunch humans regularly, even pulling them from small boats on the Nile River and spurting up to 50 yards onto land to pull down slow runners.

If you end up as an appealing morsel for a crocodile, you will be grabbed by unshakably powerful jaws. As with alligators, crocs can't chew. Having taken hold, they will then rotate rapidly along the length of their axis until the part of you they are tenaciously holding rips off. You may not feel pain yet, but you will feel the gush of your blood from the hole where a part of you was recently attached. If your arm or leg was small, an excellent possibility when compared to the appetite of the croc, the crocodile will be back for more. They, in fact, are fond of tucking food away under water for a snack later. If you happen to be tough, your storage for later consumption softens you up for added delectableness and easier dismemberment.

Moral: The only safe crocodile lives somewhere you aren't.

Cursed by Curare

"Our final experience, like our first, is conjectural. We move between two darknesses."

—E. M. Forster, 1927.

Strychnos toxifera! The name itself should give you an idea of the lethal possibilities of curare, one of the deadliest vegetable poisons on earth. Harmless if swallowed, all of the parts of this climbing vine of Central America and northern South America will exude a dark, aromatic, resinous goop that usually brings fatal results if it gets injected into you. The Orinoco Indians inject it into their victims by tipping their arrowheads and darts in the stuff. Theoretically, curare could also cause your death if you rubbed it into an open wound, but it would take a lot. Similar plants with the same effects grow in Peru and nearby countries. Medical science renders curare into a pure form used in lung surgery, in exacting amounts, to paralyze patients in order to put them on a respirator for the duration of the surgical procedures.

Once inside your body, curare begins its poisonous job of paralysis first on your eyelids and then the rest of your face. Within seconds you won't be able to swallow or even lift your head. Soon your diaphragm will stop working and you will find it extremely difficult to breathe. Your pulse will drop like a rock from a cliff. You will turn a ghastly shade of blue and your dramatic contortions as you attempt to draw breath will soon cease. The series of events surrounding your death occur so quickly that an antidote, even if one existed, would have no time to work.

Moral: Never give offense to the Orinoco.

The Shocking Truth: Electric Eel

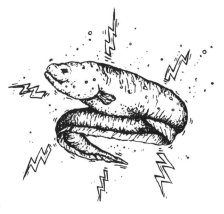

*"Rich man and poor move
side by side toward the limit
of death."*
  –Pindar, Fifth Century BC.

Though decidedly eel-like in appearance, electric eels (*Electrophorus electricus*), growing to 10 feet in length and up to 90 pounds in weight, are not true eels but fishes of shallow freshwater in Brazil, Colombia, Peru and perhaps surrounding countries. Not even a normal fish, electric eels breathe air and will drown if held underwater for 15 minutes or so, something you most assuredly do not want to do to one. For a short distance behind their heads you'll find all their vital organs, and after that a long stretch of electricity-producing tissue. Discharges of electricity from eels have been measured at 650 volts, and far less can end your life.

These creatures surround themselves with an electric field with which they navigate and sense their prey, a process that becomes more and more important to eels as they mature and lose what little eyesight they possess. They stun their prey, then consume the fishy meal while it's still alive. Eels have no interest in dead fish. They cannot control their voltage, but they can control the number of pulses of electricity they discharge. Pulses start from a point about one-fifth the way tailward from the head and run the length of its body to end at the tail. Contact with an electric eel may prove fatal, your heart stopped by the charge, and you can be knocked unconscious more than 20 feet away while you're in the water with one.

Moral: *Some people get more of a charge out of life than they
        ever expected.*

Eliminated by Elephant

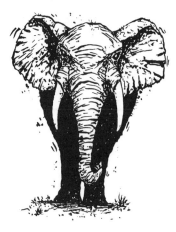

*"Dust thou art, and unto
dust thou shalt return."*
 —*Genesis 3:19.*

Once, more than 350 kinds of elephants roamed with relative tranquility over the face of the earth, not bothered by much, not bothering much. Today only two species remain: the African elephant and the Asiatic or Indian elephant. Entirely vegetarian, they daily consume vast quantities of grasses and leaves, fruits and small twigs, as much as 400 pounds per 24 hours, which they grind with four large teeth before swallowing. Social by nature, they live and move in herds with strong family ties broken only by adult bulls who leave the herd of cows and calves to lead solitary lives, returning for brief tempestuous visits during the mating season.

An adult African elephant male (*Loxodonta africana*) may stand above 10 feet at the shoulder and weigh in at more than six tons. His tusks, elongated incisor teeth, grow his whole life and have been known to reach 10 feet in length and 230 pounds each in weight. He can run at better than 20 miles per hour for long periods of time. Gentle by nature, he can be pushed beyond the endurance of his massive patience. An enraged bull elephant (maybe he has been teased too much or maybe he just has a bad attitude) will not be deterred from utterly insuring you are dead.

He will taste the you-scented air with his trunk, swinging it from side to side and then straight out toward you while his broad ears spread wide to guide every tiny bit of your sounds into his ear canals. His barely useful eyes will glisten wetly as he dances an awkward shuffle, rolling his weight from side to side. Before you realize he has started to charge, dust billows around his chest and front legs as all appearance of awkwardness suddenly dissolves into forward motion accompanied by a shrill and heart-stopping blast. If your heart starts again and fear allows you to run, your dash will cover little ground before his trunk wraps around your waist and you are lifted high over the bull's head. (Note: If he happens to spear you with a tusk, it will be an accident, but he won't care.) The thump of your body smashing with terrific force into the ground will probably end all interest you have in your own death, but your ruin has only begun. Pressing you firmly into the soil, he'll use his trunk to tear you raggedly into approximately two halves. Each half will be systematically stomped until no bone remains unbroken. At last satisfied the elephant will raise his trunk in a final trumpet of glorious victory. Later you will easily assume the shape of whatever vessel is chosen to carry away the pulp that was once a human being.

Moral: *Never joke around with anything more than 10 times your size.*

Finalized by Frog

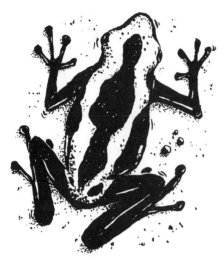

"Even the bold will fly when they see Death drawing in close enough to end their life."

—*Sophocles, c. 442 BC.*

Quite a few members of the South and Central American frog families of Atelopidae and Dendrobatidae are the most poisonous of the world's amphibians, especially the latter, the arrow-poison frogs (sometimes called poison-dart frogs). Most frog and toad skin has some degree of poison in it (see BAFFLED BY BOUGA TOAD), but nothing as potent as the arrow-poison frogs whose skin may actually contain one of the most potent biotoxins in the animal kingdom. Not much is known about the vitality of frog poison since human volunteers for scientific experiments related to why and how fast you die are hard to come by. What seems to happen is this: you get frog poison inside you and your heart speeds up until it's going so fast it runs out of gas and stops. Convulsions may add a touch of interest to your final moments.

Small and brightly colorful and reportedly dangerous to casually handle, these amphibians are carefully gathered by South American Indians who are fond of roasting poison-arrow frogs on sticks over an open fire. The poison which drips off the frying frog is collected and concocted into a potion that the Indians use to coat their arrow tips and blow darts to increase their chances of a kill while hunting. Some of the species of arrow-poison frogs have skin so poisonous the Indians simply pin the creature to the forest floor and rub the point of their weapons along the backs of the frogs. Thus the name. And thus another reason to stay on friendly terms with as many fellow earthlings as possible.

Moral: Look but don't touch.

Flattened by Funnel Web Spider

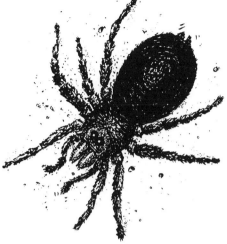

*"When we are dead, rugs are
no thicker than a quick-thorn
bed."*
  —Theognis, Six Century BC.

Australia's funnel web spiders (*Atrax robustus*) are large and aggressive, relatives to tarantulas, but, unlike tarantulas who have a relatively mild-to-humans venom, funnel web spiders pack a potent punch, enough to drop you in your tracks. The spiders are glossy black on top and velvety black on the bottom. A close look at their bottoms might reveal a few red hairs, but if you're close enough to see them you're certainly close enough to deserve a bite. Females, larger than males, might grow to as much as two inches across. And, yep, they build funnel-shaped webs like burrows under logs and rocks, stumps and dense vegetation. As with all tarantula-type spiders, the funnel web spider possesses fangs that hang down vertically, a characteristic they compensate for by raising up on their hind legs and striking like a snake. The fangs are 4 to 5 mm long and strong enough to penetrate your fingernail or your toenail, making removal of the spider from your body sometimes a problem.

You're going to feel a lot of pain from the bite, due at least as much to the power of the "strike" as to the venom itself. Within about 20 minutes, however, the pain should spread through your entire body. Another five minutes should produce high blood pressure, rapid heart rate and increased body temperature. Within two hours you ought to be sweating, drooling and crying, which are associated with diarrhea and uncontrollable, weird muscle movements. About this time you'll either start to recover or your lungs will have filled with fluid so you'll drown to death in your own body juices.

Moral: You may think it's funnel, but the joke's on you.

Held Up by Gila Monster

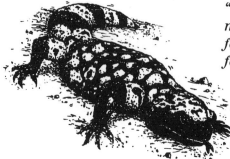

"To die completely, a person must not only forget but be forgotten, and he who is not forgotten is not dead."
–Samuel Butler, c. 1902.

About 3,000 species of lizards are known today, most of them harmless to humans, and only two species venomous, despite plenty of mythology to the contrary, and therefore potentially lethal via poison: the beaded lizards and the Gila monsters, both of the genus *Heloderma*.

While the venom glands of snakes are above their upper jaws, the venom glands of these lizards are in their lower jaws and not connected to their teeth (as in snakes). These lizards must grab hold with their strong jaw muscles and chew the venom into the wound they make. To compensate for the lack of a venom injection system, these lizards use stubborn stick-to-it-ness: once they bite, they hold on with great tenacity despite vigorous attempts to dislodge them.

Gila (hee-lah) monsters live quiet and peaceful lives, hunting at night throughout the southwestern United States and Mexico and growing to almost two feet in length. They are essentially black with smears of yellow and pink. Carrying primarily a neurotoxin in their venom, Gila monsters would not cause much pain when they bite except they hang on so tight and chew so hard. They never bite humans unless they are messed with, at which time they are capable of pivoting rapidly on their hind legs and lashing out with incredible speed.

If they work enough venom into the wound they've created on your hand or foot, you'll feel pain and see some swelling. You may feel numb and weak. You'll feel your heart speed up. You'll probably vomit, feel dizzy and have increasing difficulty breathing. Bitten humans often survive, but if you don't it will be because you are not breathing enough to stay alive.

Moral: Catch your breath, but don't catch lizards.

Grabbed by Gorilla

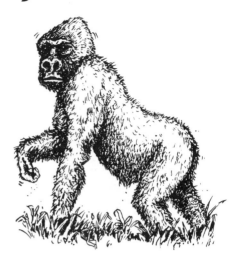

*"Any man's death diminishes
me, because I am involved in
mankind; and therefore
never send to know for whom
the bell tolls; it tolls for thee."*
–John Donne, 1624.

Members of the group called "great apes" are divided into chimpanzees (*Pan*), orangutans (*Pongo*) and the greatest of all, gorillas (*Gorilla*). Both Mountain and Lowland gorillas are found only in equatorial Africa where, although shorter than most men and women, they grow to outweigh humans by several hundred pounds, with armspans that may exceed nine feet. With stupendous strength and extraordinary intelligence, their ability to maim and ruin is more than matched by their quiet and gentle spirits, as is true of all the great apes. Able to destroy just about anything, gorillas are satisfied with a ferocious glare, a mighty bellow and a few thumps on their massive chests. They will charge you in a most realistic fashion, but physical contact with humans ranks among the rarest of incidences. You'll have to work very hard if you want to be killed by a gorilla.

Gorillas live most of their lives with four extremities on the ground, their two feet and the knuckles of their two hands. They perform their bluff charges that way, and almost everything so confronted turns and runs. Should you wade in with fists flying, you might be able to generate a devastating sideways swat or a tremendous bite from a large mouth with giant teeth and powerful jaw muscles. The gorilla will then tend to withdraw. If you are conscious and able, you could counter-attack the gorilla's counter of your attack, and possibly get annihilated, a fate you would infinitely deserve.

Moral: You can't judge a gorilla by its cover.

Gobbled by Great White Shark

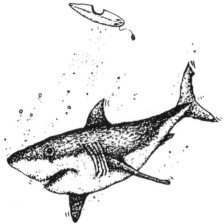

"What good can come from meeting death with tears?... If a man is sorry for himself, he doubles death."
—Euripides, c. 414 BC.

Who knows what may lurk in the dark of the deeps? At least 300 species of sharks have been identified, ranging in size at maturity from six inches to almost 50 feet (see TORN APART BY TIGER SHARK and BULLIED BY BULL SHARK). But teeth have been found, the same teeth that grow in the mouth of great white sharks, that measured five inches long. Such teeth fell from the mouths of a white shark that had grown to 100 feet in length. No shark that size has ever been recorded, but the teeth were not fossils!

Dark blue, gray, gray-green, even brown on top, great white sharks (*Carcharodon carcharias*) are only white on the bottom half. With no bones, just cartilage, and virtually no brain, white sharks are huge stretches of death-dealing muscle, the evolutionary pinnacle of a water-borne killing "machine." At maximum weights that near two tons, these sharks tend to kill and swallow large things: seals and sea lions, salmon, tuna, dolphins and great turtles and, now and then, a human. Totally fearless, great whites are the only sharks, the only fish, who will lift their eyes above the water to spot prey. To a great white shark, a human kicking along the surface of the ocean, especially on a surf board, is just another tasty morsel, something that looks sort of like some of their regular food. They seem to develop a taste for, or at least do not mind the taste of, humans (see the movie *Jaws*).

Their attacks are sudden, swift and terrifying: one huge bite from a huge mouth full of huge teeth. Then they back off and wait until their food bleeds to death. Sharks, in general, detest a struggle, and they are magnificently patient. Take all the time you want to die.

Moral: Sometimes tasting good is more important than good tastes.

Gutted by Grizzly

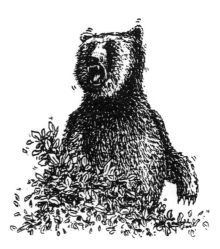

"Death is not anything... It's the absence of presence, nothing more... the endless time of never coming back... a gap you can't see, and when the wind blows through it, it makes no sound."
    – Tom Stoppard, 1967.

For thousands of years the great brown bears ruled North America from the Bering Strait to northern Mexico. Now they hide in Alaska and western Canada and in a few wilderness areas of the western United States, subdued by the guns and the greed of humans.

Growing to over 1,000 pounds in weight, inland brown bears, the grizzlies (*Ursus arctos horribilis*), are immense mounds of muscle that can run at better than 35 miles an hour. A large hump on their shoulders distinguishes the "griz" from all other bears. They possess huge feet with nonretractable claws and huge omnivorous appetites appeased on a daily basis by about 80 percent vegetables and fruit. The other 20 percent of their diet is meat.

Grizzly bears attack humans seldom and most often because they feel threatened. But, on rare occasions, a bear will attack for no apparent reason except perhaps a quick and easy snack. Although they appear most ferocious in paintings where the artist depicts them on their hind feet swapping powerfully at some poor primate, grizzly bears spend most of their lives on four feet, and they charge on four feet. Their claws are primarily for gathering food and secondarily for taking swipes at things. Their teeth are for killing and tearing off hunks of meat for consumption.

The best way to encourage a grizzly bear to attack is to run. Giving chase is one of their chief sources of entertainment. They can run fast for a long time. As soon as you get caught, remember they also enjoy wrestling, possibly because they always win. So playing dead often, but not always, discourages the bear who leaves looking for more fun, and fighting back encourages the bear to fight. Grizzly bears will cheat, biting relentlessly, especially your head and neck. Once you're dead, the bear may or may not eat you, depending on hunger. If it decides to eat, it will likely start with your guts, the most tender and juicy part of you. Either way, you lose.

Moral: If there's no chance to win, don't play.

Hammered by Hammerhead

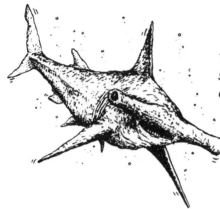

"A man's dying is more the survivors' affair than his own."

–Thomas Mann, 1924.

Of all the shark species of earth (see GOBBLED BY GREAT WHITE SHARK) only 21 species have been well documented to kill a human. Of those 21, the four species listed in this book (great white, tiger, bull, hammerhead), at least according to some experts, are the ones most likely to kill a human. Of those four, none is more regularly unpredictable than the great hammerhead shark (*Sphyrna tubes*), the weird looking fish with its eyes at either end of its hammer-shaped head. Despite the seemingly awkward placement of its jaws beneath the "hammer," hammerheads are precise killers and considered dangerous at all times. Like most sharks, hammerheads have gill slits but no way to flap their gills, so in order to breathe, they stay in motion, forcing oxygen-rich water across their gills, all their lives. This may explain in part their tendency to be irritable. Hammerheads, at a maximum length of around 14 feet, can be carrying a load of irritability.

The fear sharks induce in humans is not reflected in their kill rate, their attacks being fatal about 30 times a year worldwide. If you are confronted by a hammerhead, or any shark, and you suddenly discover you want to live, face the shark and stay as calm as possible. If the shark approaches close enough, try kicking, punching and gouging its eyes, none of which will hurt the shark in the least but some of which might discourage it. Screaming sometimes, it has been reported, might make you feel better. If you are alone, swimming away as fast as you can is utterly useless.

Moral: Always swim in shark-infested waters with someone who swims a lot slower than you.

Hung Up on Hantavirus

"Though it be in the power of the weakest arm to take away life, it is not in the strongest to deprive us of death."

—Thomas Browne, 1642.

Carried in rodent urine, and probably in mousy feces and saliva, hantavirus can become airborne through misting of the urine or in dust from dried feces and nests. The virus has been found predominantly in deer mice, but also in pinyon mice and chipmunks. So far, no known transmission of the germs has occurred between insects and humans or humans and humans. You can sleep on the ground near a nest, outside your tent, or camp sloppily and attract sick rodents to your campsite. Then you breathe in the mist or dust and have the virus take up residence in your lungs regardless of your age, weight, height, gender or ethnic background.

You'll start with fever and muscle aches and think, rats, you've contracted some kind of flu. More symptoms develop, such as stomach pain and nausea, that fail to alter your first self-diagnosis. You may have a cough, headache and, sometimes, itchy inflamed eyes. But then, wham, the sudden onset of severe difficulty breathing as your lungs start to fill with fluid. The problem gets progressively worse until you can breathe no more.

On the really interesting side, so far, no known virus has ever caused this specific type of illness in the past. You could be one of a few.

Moral: Never rat on your friends.

Too Hot To Handle: Heat Stroke

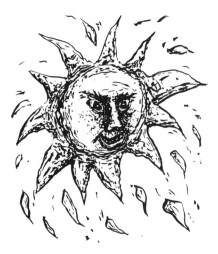

*"Death is but an instant, life
a long torment."*
–Bernard Joseph Saurin, 1768.

If your body produces heat faster than it sheds heat (see THE BIG CHILL: HYPOTHERMIA), you can cook yourself to death in your own juices, a condition called heat stroke, or hyperthermia. Your internal fluid level works more than anything else to keep you cool, so getting dehydrated ranks as the primary pathway to heat stroke. You can dehydrate (lose internal water) outdoors in several ways: sweat, peeing, pooping, even breathing. The hotter the air is and the harder you exercise, the faster you lose water. If you're used to the heat, you can lose up to one-and-a-half quarts in one hour while doing something strenuous.

To be officially heat stroked, your core body temperature has to reach 105°F, but before that you'll feel hot, tired, headachey and maybe dizzy and nauseous, a condition known as heat exhaustion. You can take a break, drink water, find some shade and take a dip if a lake or stream lies nearby, or you can keep pushing yourself. By the time you reach 105°F, your brain will have altered significantly from normal, leaving you bizarrely different from the person you used to be. Your skin will be very red and very hot to the touch. Your skin may also be dry, but in outdoorsy types skin is usually still wet with sweat. Bystanders will probably find your hallucinations and seizures fascinating. Unless someone who cares about you is around to cool you off by pouring on lots of water, fanning and massaging, your body systems will begin to shut down one by one until you no longer function as a human being.

Moral: Hydrate or die!

Hassled by Helminth

"Those most like the dead are those most loath to die."
                                        —La Fontaine, c. 1688.

Helminths are worms that take up residence inside a human being. They are found around the world, primarily in tropical and subtropical countries, and are estimated to live in the guts of approximately one out of every three human earthlings. Most of the species of intestinal worms, and there are many, don't reproduce while inside you, but you can provide habitat for quite a few of these stringy creatures for long periods of time and never know it. Obviously, not everyone dies from internal helminth infestations, but thousands do every year, mostly in less developed countries and mostly children.

You can swallow the eggs of the worms, which subsequently hatch inside you, when you eat meat or vegetables infected by some types of these worms. You can be bitten by insects that are carrying some of the worms. Some of them can actually "worm" their way through your skin when you're swimming in infected fresh water.

Roundworms (*Ascaris lumbricoides*) are the most popular parasitic worms worldwide with residences well established in a staggering one out of every four humans. This helminth is transmitted by ingestion of their eggs, which probably got into your vegetables from contaminated soil. After the eggs hatch in your small intestines, the larvae crawl through the mucosa to enter your bloodstream, eventually ending up in your lungs where they rupture through into your alveoli and squirm up your trachea where you swallow them a second time for a return trip to your intestines. Mature roundworms will live out their lives quite happily in your intestines, reaching a foot or more in length, mating and laying more eggs and sucking your blood. You don't feel a thing unless so many of the worms get inside they suck you to death. At least you'll deposit the fresh eggs with your next defecation, giving you the opportunity to spread the wealth around.

Moral: It pays to not get too eggs-cited.

Tea for Tomb: Water Hemlock

"Nobody knows, in fact, what death is, nor whether to man it is not perchance the greatest of all blessings; yet people fear it as if they surely knew it to be the worst of evils."

—Socrates, c. 399 b.c.

Shortly after Socrates, the infinitely brilliant Greek philosopher, uttered two of the most important words ever uttered, "Know thyself," he was forced to drink tea brewed from *Cicuta maculata* or perhaps a related species, a plant called water hemlock. The year was 399 BC. Apparently his innovative philosophies were deemed subversive by the State.

Water hemlock grows, as you would expect, along the banks of waterways or in wet meadows throughout North America. It bears, in addition to hemlock, such names as children's bane, beaver poison, death-of-man, poison parsnip and false parsley. A member of the parsnip or carrot family, it stands tall with hollow stems and a bundle of short rootstocks that exude an oily yellow juice when cut. Its leaves alternate and are pinnate, with two to three leaflets that are narrow, toothed and pointy. flowers are white and small, blossoming in flat-topped umbrella-like clusters, like a carrot in bloom. The entire plant, but especially the roots and young plants in spring, are poisonous. A full grown adult can be killed by one bite of root, and children have died from simply using the hollow stems as peashooters. The poison is resin-like cicutoxin, a toxin that acts on the central nervous system of the victim. Many death-by-plant experts consider water hemlock to be the most poisonous plant in the North Temperate Zone.

Within 30 minutes of consuming water hemlock you will vomit and have a convulsion or two. You may feel better after puking, but the plant only wills you into a false sense of security. Soon your heart rate will speed up, your pupils will dilate and you'll sweat like you just ran a marathon in July in southern Georgia. You'll begin to froth at the mouth and jerk violently in severe seizures. You'll probably experience extraordinary stomach pain, vomit a time or two more, slip into delirium and stop breathing for a few minutes now and then. Paralysis will take over, and soon you'll stop breathing forever.

Moral: Know thy water-related plants.

Harassed by Hippopotamus

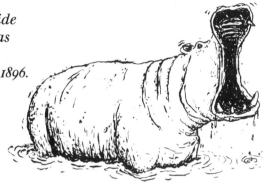

*"It is death that is the guide
of our life, and our life has
no goal but death."
—Maurice Maeterlinck, 1896.*

Once they wobbled fatly over the entire continent of Africa, but now hippopotamuses, "river horses," stake out their territories in relatively few regions in shallow rivers with open grassland nearby. They are prevalent, for instance, in the Zambezi River of Zimbabwe. They stick to the water during the day, nibbling water plants, and come out at night to graze on land plants. Hippos require an average of between 50 and 90 pounds of food per day to sustain their 3,000 to 8,000 pound bodies. Although they clump together in sociable herds, the encroachment of any human into their territory typically causes an attack by a dominant male or a nursing mother. Hippos kill more humans every year than all the lions, elephants and buffaloes of Africa combined.

In the water they are especially aggressive, easily "swimming" down any human and chomping small boats in half. They actually swim rather poorly and sink to the bottom immediately when the water deepens over their heads. They run along the bottom of rivers, staying underwater for up to five minutes. On land they are capable of reaching speeds of 45 miles per hour when aroused.

A hippo yawns to warn you. Inside that monstrously gaping mouth are sharp canine teeth guided by powerful jaw muscles, but none of a hippo's diet consists of meat. One chomp with no swallowing will usually satisfy the hippo, and easily satisfies the coroner who is required to list your cause of death.

Moral: The wise heed warnings.

Hounded by Hyena

"Life does not cease to be funny when people die any more than it ceases to be serious when people laugh."
                                        —George Bernard Shaw, 1913.

Frequently thought of as cowards slinking just outside the light of your campfire, eaters of carrion with demented laughs piercing dark African nights, hyenas are relatively intelligent, strict meat-eaters and, even though they do scavenge, capable of aggressive attacks, singly and in teams, on very-much-alive humans.

With wide grins and backs that slant noticeably toward the rear, hyenas (collectively called Hyaenidae) appear like canines designed by a committee of politicians, but actually have more attributes of cats than dogs. Their range, once throughout most of Europe, Asia and Africa, is now limited to Africa, India and the Near East. Equipped with some of the most powerful jaws in the animal kingdom, hyenas can snap bones that defy the teeth of more formidable looking mammals. And spotted hyenas of Africa do have a horrendous and spine-tingling "laugh."

Hyenas have nasty dining habits which include a marked tendency to eat and run: they'll rush up to you while you doze unprotected, rip off a significant portion of your face (their favorite target) and dash into the bush while still swallowing. If you are small enough, a hyena will grab an arm or leg and bound away with you in tow. Never deeply committed to munching humans, hyenas are extremely dedicated to opportunity eating, creatures upon whom you should never turn your back.

Moral: The one who laughs last, laughs best.

The Big Chill: Hypothermia

"The grave's a fine and private place, but none, I think, do there embrace."

—Andrew Marvell, 1650.

From the food you eat your body manufactures energy for living, with heat as a by-product. You produce so much heat your blood would boil several times a day if you didn't naturally and involuntarily shed the heat through cooling mechanisms: radiation, evaporation, convection and conduction (see Too Hot To Handle: Heat Stroke). If you expose yourself to the cooling mechanisms, you'll keep on shedding heat even when you aren't producing very much, and the warmth at the core of your body (normally about 98.6°F) will start to drop. A drop in core body temperature is called hypothermia.

Although medical science describes hypothermia as a core body temperature of 95°F or lower, things happen before you reach that point. The first thing to happen is a loss of mental acuity: you get stupid. Signs of stupidity include not putting on raingear when it starts to rain, not eating when you're hungry, not drinking water even though you know you need a lot and not camping when it gets too dark to see the trail. You may have trouble with fine motor activities like zipping up your parka. At around 95°F you'll start to shiver. The shivering will get worse and worse, and you'll have trouble doing gross motor activities like walking, so you sit down or lie down and keep losing heat to the environment. Suddenly the shivering stops because you no longer have enough energy to shiver. You've run out of gas. Your heart rate and breathing rate will slow down and down, and your muscles will begin to grow rigid. You won't care because you're stupid. Some hypothermic humans who have been re-warmed from being this cold claim they began to feel comfortable, warm and sleepy. Soon you'll lose consciousness.

You can live for a long time, days maybe, in this profound hypothermic state, but eventually your heart will stop. If anyone ever finds your body, you'll look and feel like a human popsicle.

Moral: Intelligence is only skin deep, but stupid goes clear to the bone.

Jumped by Jellyfish

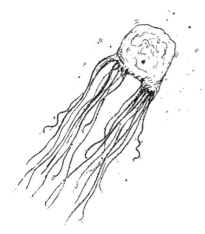

"Do not rejoice over anyone's death; remember that we all must die."
–*Ecclesiasticus* 7:7.

Jellyfish belong to the phylum Coelenterata, the coelenterates, which include sea anemones, corals and hydroids (see MANGLED BY MAN-OF-WAR). From almost microscopic to the giant lion's mane (*Cyanea capillata*) with a body over seven feet in diameter and tentacles dangling down more than 100 feet, true jellyfish (globes of "jelly" with "strings" hanging from it) drift on the sea of life in all the oceans of earth. Some cause humans no harm at all. Some cause humans mild pain and some cause screaming pain. A few cause an agonizing death.

Jellyfish work this way: Their tentacles are covered in specialized stinging organelles called nematocysts, which are contained in specialized cells called cnidoblasts. Each cnidoblast has a cnidocil, a "trigger," that activates the cell when something, such as a human, touches it. When touched, a "trapdoor" called an operculum flies open and a spring-loaded, microscopic, barbed venom sac plunges into, let's say, an arm. One swipe of the arm through the tentacles of a jellyfish can stimulate thousands to hundreds of thousands of nematocysts to fire out their venomous daggers. No jellyfish attacks humans. They just automatically sting everything they bump into, hoping it will turn out to be food.

Common from the Philippines to Australia, the box jellyfish (*Chironex fleckeri*), sometimes mistakenly called a sea wasp (which is another dangerous jellyfish, *Carybdea marsupialis*), carries a venom among the earth's most deadly to humans, sometimes killing in 30 seconds! Indeed, this is one of the world's most lethal poisons. If you have time, you'll notice profound muscle spasms and muscular and respiratory paralysis. You won't notice, but your blood pressure will drop. Suddenly your heart will stop. It's the Deep Six, and you're food for the crabs.

Moral: Just because something is smaller than you doesn't mean you should push it around.

The Big Trip: Jimsonweed

*"...wisdom says: We must die,
and seeks how to make us die
well."*
–Miquel de Unamuno, 1924.

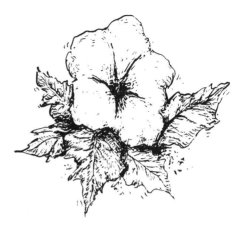

Shamans supposedly brewed a tea of jimsonweed (*Datura stramonium*), or a similar *Datura* species, and sipped their way into an altered state of consciousness in which secrets of the spirit world were revealed. History does not reveal how many shamans became permanent spirit world residents via jimsonweed, but you can rest assured the whole plant, especially the roots, leaves and seeds, contains hyoscyamine, a poison of the highest quality, a doorway to death through which many humans have passed. A lush green plant at maturity, the juices and wilted leaves hold the most toxin as soldiers sent to Jamestown, VA, in 1666 discovered when they ran out of food and ate the berries and collapsed by the score. From Jamestown weed the named was corrupted to jimsonweed, also called Devil's trumpet (the white or purple flowers are trumpet-shaped), stinkweed (it doesn't smell great), thorn apple (the berries are prickly) and mad apple (if you survive a sampling, you may report unpleasant hallucinations).

What you can expect several hours after consumption includes headache, dizziness, thirst (which can be extreme), a dry burning feeling in your skin, dilated pupils and a corresponding blurring of vision, perhaps blindness, delirium and manic activity, drowsiness, a weak pulse, a few seizures, coma and, very likely, death. Some experts claim jimsonweed causes more poisonings than any other plant in the United States.

Moral: Some trips are worth the cost, and some aren't.

Killed by Killer Whale

"Pity is for the living, envy is for the dead."

—*Mark Twain, 1897.*

Communal creatures, killer whales (*Orcinus orca*) live in tight knit herds (or pods) with individual IQs that equal or surpass the great apes. Ranging from the Arctic to the Antarctic, largest of the dolphins, warm-blooded and air-breathing, black with attractive smears of white, they grow to over 30 feet in length and undoubtedly deserve their name: they feed regularly on warm-blooded animals (seals, penguins, porpoises, smaller dolphins), their favored food by far. Inside their Herculean jaws are conical teeth up to two inches across at the base. Speedy of fin, they can swim down any of their chosen food sources. When driven by hunger, they will rise six or eight feet out of the water to spot a meal on a beach or ice floe and throw themselves well up onto land or ice to reach intended prey. They have been watched repeatedly battering floes in attempts to dislodge seals. Other whales, often substantially larger than killer whales, have been known to launch themselves onto land (where they suffocate, unable to expand their lungs due to their massive body weight) in order to escape the onslaught of a pod of starving *orcas*.

From centuries of human observation of these mighty animals a most astounding fact emerges: not once has a killer whale ever been proven to kill a human. There are incidents in which killer whales "appeared" to attack a human, such as flopping up on ice where a man or woman was standing. But these cases are almost undoubtedly examples of mistaken identity. The whales thought they were going for a seal. It is theoretically possible to be killed if you dive into a pod of hungry killer whales after smearing seal blubber all over yourself. That would definitely rate as an interesting way to die.

Moral: A whale of a good time is more an attitude than an event.

Creamed by Komodo Dragon

*"Death always comes too
early or too late."*
    –English Proverb.

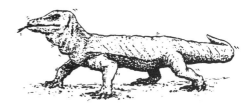

Komodo lies about 240 miles east of Bali in Indonesia, a desolate, volcanic, "moon-surfaced" island, home to the largest lizard living on earth, the fabulous and fierce Komodo dragon. Only here and on five neighboring islands do there be dragons. Dark gray and scaly with flabby necks, short snouts and large mouths filled with small daggers, Komodo dragons are up to 10 feet in length, up to 500 pounds in weight, and up to no good when hungry or aggravated. Extraordinary athletes, they can easily run down the swiftest human runner and swim down the swiftest human swimmer. They can dig fast, climb fast and eat fast, and their diet consists largely of meat: wild buffaloes, wild deer, wild pigs, wild goats and wild humans dumb enough to get too near. They also eat each other, a habit that keeps baby Komodo dragons pretty much in the tops of trees for the first couple of years of life.

Nearly deaf and nearly blind, these dragons can smell dinner up to four miles away with a favoring breeze. Unless an impenetrable fence separates you from these giant lizards at feeding time, you are dead meat... or soon to be dead meat. Usually solitary, they team up at meal time, when there's enough to go around, and easily polish off a whole human in 15 or 20 minutes. Dead or alive, Komodo dragons don't care. They've even been known to raid graveyards, exhuming and devouring human corpses.

Moral: Good fences do not guarantee good neighbors.

Latched Onto by Leech

"Why is it that we rejoice at a birth and grieve at a funeral? It is because we are not the person involved."
                                        —Mark Twain, 1894.

Evolving from the same source as the earthworm, 650 or so species of leeches come in a variety of colors, shapes and sizes, all of which are worm-like, swimming, slimy, blood-sucking lifeforms. Unlike most blood-suckers of the world, leeches carry no germs transmissible to humans. They'll undulate over to a disturbance in the water where they congregate and explore the disturbing thing with their puckered mouths. Leeches seek out warmth, the source of their favorite food: mammalian blood. If the thing meets the meal plan, they attach with a rear sucker and start gnawing through with the front sucker, which contains three serrated jaws formed in sort of a three-pointed star pattern. They'll suck until they've added as much as nine times their starting weight. Little leeches suck out a little blood. Huge leeches suck out a lot. Little leeches don't hurt much and, in fact, you may not know they're feeding. Huge leeches hurt a lot.

The hugest leech of all is the secretive giant leech (*Haementeria ghilianii*), last studied a few years ago in the marshy land of French Guiana. A greenish-brown wob of goo, giant leeches grow to 18 inches. One giant leech could feed to the point where you got kind of woozy. Two could probably feed until you passed out. Three might kill you. But nobody knows for sure because it's difficult to get volunteers to put up with the pain and blood loss. Should you choose to investigate, your death could be valuable to scientific research.

Widely known throughout Southeast Asia, a small leech (*Dinobdella ferox*) prefers to crawl up the nasopharyngeal (nose and throat) passage and feed in the back of the throat of mammals, including humans. Theoretically, enough of them could slime in to choke you. Nobody knows about that for sure either.

Moral: There's a sucker born every minute.

Leaped on by Leopard

"It is better that we live ever so miserably than die in glory."
—Euripides, c. 405 BC.

Even though these cats are divided into at least 15 "races" from southern Africa north into Russia, from Malaysia to Israel, from below sea level to 18,000 feet, they are all basically the leopard (*Panthera pardis*), one of if not the most widely distributed large mammal of earth. Among all the cats of the world that regularly kill and consume humans, the leopard holds a special place. Smallest of the man-eaters, reaching maybe 120 pounds, the leopard is by weight the most powerful, able to drag a 150 pound man four miles after the kill, and, despite its size, the most intelligent. Leopards, say the experts, know what you're thinking. With no cat is the human hunter more likely to become the hunted... and the devoured. Single leopards that have become dedicated to man-eating have ended the lives of as many as 400 men, women and children.

Extraordinarily keen of nightsight, leopards sneak up in utter silence to leap, always, for the throat of their victims, be it antelope, buffalo or you. From behind, your neck will most likely be broken by the powerful bite. From the front, your windpipe will be torn out, resulting in death by suffocation. Either way four long canines are driven in faster than a carpenter could drive in nails with a nailgun. And leopards have the extremely nasty habit of ripping repeatedly with their hind claws, shredding with those needle-tipped daggers until your guts are strewn along the ground, a problem with which you will have no concern since you'll be close enough to death by then to not care.

Moral: Discretion is the better part of remaining in one piece.

Laid Low by Leptospirosis

"Death hath a thousand doors to let out life."
—Philip Massinger, 1655.

Members of an order of slender, spiral, microscopic organisms, belonging to the class Schizomycetes, *Leptospira* are spirochetes with hooked or curved ends, and leptospirosis is the disease these organisms cause once they get inside humans.

Although infected wild animals, including some frogs and snakes, show no signs of the disease, they shed the spirochetes freely in their urine. Human cases, usually less than 100 each year which appear in the United States, are most often acquired from contact with contaminated water, and sometimes from contact with soil. Swallowing is the primary way *Leptospira* get inside people, but the organisms can "worm" in through abraded skin and through the mucous membranes of eye and mouth. You can also get sick from contacting infected animal blood and tissues.

Leptospirosis appears throughout tropical and temperate regions of the world, and is most commonly seen in Southeast Asia and some areas of Latin America. Recent cases have been brought back from lower Central America.

Numerous types of *Leptospira* exist, but the signs and symptoms they produce in humans are much the same. One to two weeks (can be as long as three) after becoming host to the spirochetes, the first of two phases of the disease begins. Phase one lasts four to seven days and shows up in many patients as fever, chills, headache, enlarged lymph nodes, malaise and a nonproductive cough. After a couple of days off, the disease reappears in a second phase with a lower fever and a severe headache that won't go away. A "spotty" rash sometimes appears. Muscle aches, stomach pain, nausea and vomiting can result in either or both phases. Death occurs in about five percent of the cases when the organisms work their way into your kidneys, liver or heart.

Moral: Keep your mouth shut.

Lit Up by Lightning

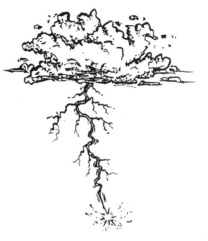

"To die with glory, if one has to die at all, is still, I think, pain for the dier."
—*Euripides, c. 455 BC.*

When warm, moist air rises rapidly to great heights, dark clouds filled with static electricity tend to form. A charge accumulates on the bottom and an opposite charge on the top of the cloud and on the ground beneath the cloud. When the difference between the charges reaches a potential greater than the ability of the air to insulate, lightning stretches out to equalize the difference. Direct current, the bolt can reach 200 million volts and 300,000 amps and a temperature of 8,000°c.

Lightning lights the skies over the earth approximately eight million times every day, roughly 100 times per second, an astounding number of discharges of electricity of which you will see very few. The bolts fly from ground to cloud, cloud to ground, cloud to cloud and within a cloud.

You can dramatically increase your opportunity to become a lightning rod by being the highest point around: on top of a mountain or open ridge, at the edge of a large body of water, out in the middle of an open field. You can add electrical attractiveness to yourself by holding onto something metal: mountain bike, ice axe, fishing pole with metal parts.

Lightning can kill you in four ways, but you won't have anything to say about it. (1) A direct strike will turn you immediately into something akin to a large potato chip. (2) Lightning can "splash" on you off of something nearby that is more attractive than you, and short-circuit your heart and breathing or (3) the ground current from a nearby strike can have the same effect on your cardiopulmonary system. (4) You can be blasted by the exploding air of a nearby strike and thrown against an object, say a tree or rock, with enough force to snuff out your life.

Moral: Always hike with someone considerably taller than you.

Lunched On by Lion

"To die is to leave off dying and do the thing once for all."
—Samuel Butler, c. 1902.

The lion (*Panthera leo*) once roamed with kingly or queenly mien over all of Africa except the densest forest and highest mountains and well north into Europe and throughout the Near East. Now it is an animal almost exclusively of the open bush and savanna, the great grasslands of Africa, never entering the jungle. Weighing in at 200 to 400 pounds and able to leap 20 feet or more in a single bound, *leo* is not the largest or most powerful cat, an honor held by the Siberian tiger, a close relative (see SLAIN BY SIBERIAN TIGER). Female lions do most of the day-to-day hunting and killing, typically at dusk, dawn and night, singling out a slow, weak individual from a herd. Aside from the occasional man-eater with an odd predilection for humans, lions prefer a juicy antelope or a toothsome wildebeest, but they have few reservations about lunching on a bipedal primate when the menu is limited. With little stamina, lions are relegated to one short burst of astounding speed. That's usually all it takes.

A dash and a leap, and the lion makes contact with your quivering flesh. A staggering blow from a forepaw of remarkable strength will be quickly followed by the sinking of long teeth into your neck. One bite and your neck snaps, and whatever interest you had in life fades like a speeding bullet. Your last movement will be a couple of involuntary and convulsive kicks. One lion will eat up to 60 pounds at one sitting, but since the pride will share you, tearing off great hunks for noisy gulps, you'll be no more than a single fast-food meal.

Moral: One who travels in the middle of herds of slower,
weaker humans, travels longer.

Licked by Lyme Disease

"You will not die because you are ill, but because you're alive."
Seneca, First Century AD.

Bacteria of the order Spirochaetales include *Borrelia burgdorferi*, a spiral-shaped organism, the cause of Lyme disease. First recognized in the area around Lyme, CT, in 1975, now at least 45 States believe the disease is transmitted by ticks in their area, the deer tick getting most of the blame. Lyme disease, or something very nearly Lyme disease, has cropped up in Europe, Asia and Australia. The bacteria live in animals, deer mice being a huge reservoir, and the ticks feed on infected blood and then pass the disease to you if you happen to be around at the appropriate time. If you remove an imbedded tick with tweezers by grabbing it gently near your skin and pulling straight out, if you do this within 48 hours after the tick bites into you, you will probably not get sick.

Lyme disease has three stages: (1) An average of seven days after the tick bite, you develop a marvelous red rash with definite borders that appears in some areas of your body to fade and reappear in other areas. With antibiotic treatment, the rash disappears altogether in several days. Without antibiotics, the rash hangs around for an average of four weeks. (2) Malaise and fatigue start from days to weeks after the bacteria get inside you, and can become severe. A low fever and muscle aches and other signs and symptoms that you might associate with a "flu-bug" manifest themselves. This can go on for weeks. (3) Your knees and other large joints start to ache with arthritis after about a year or so.

It is very, very difficult to die from Lyme disease. You have to be cursed, and the bacteria has to work its way into your heart and cause a block in the impulses that keep your heart beating and the block has to be severe enough to prevent it being corrected.

Moral: Don't get ticked off, get the tick off.

Manhandled by Mamba

"All our life is but a going out to the place of execution, to death."

–John Donne, 1619.

The mambas of Africa (black, green, western green and Jameson's), closely related to the cobras, are extremely agile and extremely fast, the fastest snakes on earth, and often extremely aggressive. If it is true that any snake will go out its way to attack a human, this is the one, especially the black mambas (*Dendroaspis polylepis*), snakes that grow to 14 feet in length with a width averaging between three and four inches. Not totally black, more outlined in black, they prefer thick grass and dense brush, making a surprise meeting with a mamba possible and potentially deadly. They can climb trees almost as fast as they slither across the ground and, to add complications to your life, mambas are most dangerous when confronted with a moving target at which they tend to thoughtlessly strike. When they arise monstrously tall, taller than the tallest grass, it is the unusual human who will simply stand still and observe.

Of all snakes, the ill effects of being bitten usually appear most rapidly after mamba bites. Sometimes referred to as "three-step" snakes, the nickname means you'll take three steps after the bite and keel over dead. It is not likely your death will occur this fast... four steps, maybe. Actually the venom, a neurotoxin, first causes, in most cases, difficulty swallowing, speaking and seeing, followed by creeping paralysis that finally affects your respiratory system until you breathe no more. How fast this happens depends, in part, on how scared you are.

Moral: It's easy to be brave when danger lies a long way off.

Mangled by Man-of-War

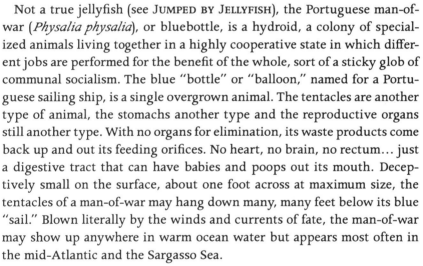

*"Death has but one terror,
that it has no tomorrow."*
—Eric Hoffer, 1954.

Not a true jellyfish (see JUMPED BY JELLYFISH), the Portuguese man-of-war (*Physalia physalia*), or bluebottle, is a hydroid, a colony of specialized animals living together in a highly cooperative state in which different jobs are performed for the benefit of the whole, sort of a sticky glob of communal socialism. The blue "bottle" or "balloon," named for a Portuguese sailing ship, is a single overgrown animal. The tentacles are another type of animal, the stomachs another type and the reproductive organs still another type. With no organs for elimination, its waste products come back up and out its feeding orifices. No heart, no brain, no rectum... just a digestive tract that can have babies and poops out its mouth. Deceptively small on the surface, about one foot across at maximum size, the tentacles of a man-of-war may hang down many, many feet below its blue "sail." Blown literally by the winds and currents of fate, the man-of-war may show up anywhere in warm ocean water but appears most often in the mid-Atlantic and the Sargasso Sea.

Swim into one of these colonies and you'll experience instant and agonizing pain. Raised welts where the tentacles struck will rise up to red heights. You may feel like a whale has beached on your chest, making it difficult to breathe. Pain may wash through your abdomen and lower back with muscle cramps extending down your legs and arms. Try to relax if you don't want to die. Being non-lethal in venom, the cause of death is most often panic and drowning.

Moral: Socialism isn't for everyone.

Misguided by Manchineel

"Death surprises us in the midst of our hopes."
— Thomas Fuller, 1732.

Old Carib Indians dipped their arrowheads in the juice in case their aim failed to reach a vital organ. Clive Cussler splashed it in the Beef Wellington to knock off almost the entire passenger list of an airline flight in *Treasure*. Early explorers, shipwrecked sailors and typical tourists have permanently succumbed to the sweet-tasting, crabapple-sized and crabapple-shaped manchineel growing in the Caribbean and around the Gulf of Mexico, including southern Florida's coastal hammocks.

Look for a small tree that sprawls near the ground with rough, warty bark and oval leaves. The flowers may be yellow or red, giving way to light-green or yellow fruit. The sap is milky. If you loaf beneath the leaves in a rain, water dripping onto your skin will give you a severe rash, probably within 30 minutes. Rub your rain-washed or sap-soaked finger in your eye and temporary blindness results. Toss the branches in a campfire and the smoke is likely to produce a romping headache and a wickedly uncomfortable eye irritation.

But eating the tasty fruit (or the leaves) is a dead giveaway. One to two hours later your lips, mouth and throat will swell, burn and blister. Stomach pain will be followed by vomiting and bloody diarrhea. Your pulse will soar and your breathing rate will follow. Your blood pressure will drop and your face will drop to the ground and before too awfully long your body will be pushing up manchineel.

Moral: Sweetness ain't necessarily goodness.

Massacred by Moccasin

"Could the Devil work my belief to imagine I could never die, I would not outlive that very thought."

— *Thomas Browne, 1642.*

Being light of bone, snakes don't fossilize very well, and it's difficult to say when they first appeared in the grand scheme of things, somewhere probably between eight and 20 million years ago. At some point along the evolutionary line the pit vipers developed their unique heat-sensitive facial pits and many of them developed rattles. Copperheads and cottonmouth water moccasins, pit vipers both, do not grow rattles, but are poisonous nonetheless. Especially poisonous is the water moccasin (genus *Agkistrodon*), rated by numerous experts as the third most deadly snake in the United States, causing more deaths than all other snakes except Eastern and Western diamondbacks (see RIPPED BY RATTLESNAKE).

An inhabitant of shallow lakes, lazy streams and swamps in the southeastern States up to southern Illinois, water moccasins grow three to six feet long with a broad head distinctly leading its dull brownish-black body through life. White lines, sometimes easy to see, sometimes not, run back from both eyes. When it opens its mouth wide, the inside looks very white and "cottony." Known for their aggressiveness, moccasins, when threatened, tend to slither rapidly toward you instead of away.

You should feel pain and see swelling not long after either or both of the long fangs sink into your flesh. If you got it in a leg or arm, your whole extremity should look relatively disgusting within an hour, and certainly within a few hours, with blood-filled blebs forming near the bite site and black-and-blue discoloration ascending toward your heart. You might feel tingling and numbness in your face and head. You might pull out of the experience in fairly healthy shape, or you might lose the arm or leg, or you might lose your blood pressure, go into shock and coma and death as your blood loses it ability to support your life.

Moral: Keep your cotton-picking hands (and feet) away from water moccasins.

Muffled by Monkshood

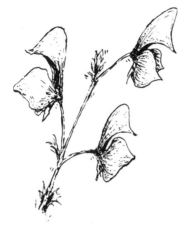

"One must take all one's life to learn how to live, and, what will perhaps make you wonder more, one must take all one's life to learn how to die."
—Seneca, First Century AD.

Throughout the Northern Hemisphere in temperate areas you'll find a perennial herbaceous plant, genus *Aconitum* and several species, with dark blue or yellow monks-hood-shaped flowers, pointy palmate leaves and a vivacious poison lurking in the whole plant, especially the leaves and roots. Looking edible, the roots have been mistaken for wild radish and consumed by humans, and the leaves have been tossed in salads. Monobasic alkaloids including aconine and aconitine can be ingested when you eat monkshood, or absorbed if the plant is rubbed on your skin. These poisons are most active before the plant flowers. Theoretically, you could persevere and rub enough into your skin to kill you, but you only have to eat very little of the plant for totally fatal results.

The early signs of your imminent death occur almost immediately: burning and tingling, maybe numbness, in the nose, throat and face followed quickly by nausea, vomiting, blurred vision and a prickly feeling in your skin. Your heart rate will grow slow and weak, and you'll feel chest pain. Sweat will pour off you just before a series of convulsions set in. Numbness will spread over your entire body, and you'll feel cold from head to toe, as if your blood has been exchanged for ice water. Right behind numbness comes an unusual combo of paralysis and severe pain, a combo that freezes your breathing muscles and your heart. Consciousness commonly prevails until the very end, and some victims have complained of "yellow-green vision" and "ringing" in the ears. Death has occurred in as little as 10 minutes.

Moral: Wear caution, and leave the hoods to the monks.

Messed Up by Moose

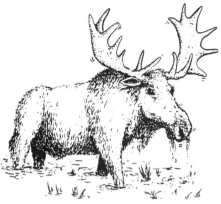

"Death is a thing of grandeur... It is a rearrangement of the world."
—*Saint-Exupery, 1942.*

Members of the deer family are ubiquitous worldwide, and come in a great variety from the very small to the very bulking. Of all the large mammals, they are usually the last to flee the encroachment of humans, indicating they are either very brave, very stubborn or not very smart. Hunted heavily in most areas, however, deer have grown reasonably afraid of humans, and retire readily when approached... most of the time.

Sharp of hoof, with a weight that might reach 1,000 pounds, with antlers (males only) that may spread to eight feet across, moose (genus *Alces*) are the largest members of the deer family and particularly easy to offend, especially in the season of the rut when bulls establish their harems and charge any intruder at the slightest provocation. Moose wounded by careless hunters regularly turn to attempt to kill the hunter. Moose moms will aggressively protect their young. On national parkland, where tourists tend to think of wild animals as not-so-wild, irate moose have been known to attack automobiles and sink small boats (moose spend a lot of their days in water) and end human lives.

Lowered head, flaring nostrils, flattened ears and bristling hair indicate moose are upset. Head down and hooves thundering across the wilderness, a bull moose charge is an impressive spectacle. They'll lead with an antler, and you'll go flying with ripped flesh and crushed bone. Once you're subdued, moose seldom hesitate to use their hooves for a few final tromps, just to make sure you understand their dislike of your trespass. Cows, and bulls too, can use their hooves to great and deadly advantage with remarkable accuracy against any target, whether it's standing, lying down or running away. You do not need to die to satisfy moose. They'll walk away while you're still breathing. But dead or alive, you're going to be a mess.

Moral: Neatness counts.

Murdered by Mosquito

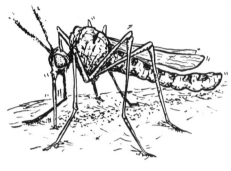

"We all labour against our own cure, for death is the cure of all diseases."
–Sir Thomas Browne, 1642.

For a long time, say 200 million years or thereabouts, the irritating whine of mosquitoes has plagued other living things on earth. Beginning life as larvae that wiggle almost invisibly in still water where 'skeeter eggs are laid, they progress to the pupal stage, frantically contorting back and forth like deranged commas, and finally to the insidious adult stage in which the females, who need blood to reproduce, go in search of prey. Both males and females can eat plant juice, but the males stick to their vegetarian diet. Females seek out anything with blood that they can stick their needle-tipped mouthparts into.

With wings whirring at 600 beats per second, with eyes that see virtually in all directions at once, they primarily follow their sense of smell to heat, lactic acid, carbon dioxide, ammonia and water vapor: signs of a warm-blooded animal.

Mosquitoes carry more diseases than any other living creatures in the entire known universe. They carry the protozoa *Plasmodia* (all four species) that cause more than 200 million new cases of malaria per year. They carry the germs for yellow fever, dengue fever and encephalitis, to name some of the most popular. Mosquitoes will make approximately 250 million humans sick this year, and over one million will die. Most of the dead were recently living in places where there is no mosquito netting, insect repellent or drug therapies against the germs. Since mosquito-borne diseases have been almost totally extinguished in the United States, you're going to have to do some traveling to die from a mosquito bite… anyplace in Central or South America, Africa or Asia should do.

Moral: The only good 'skeeter is a dead 'skeeter.

Misled by Mushroom

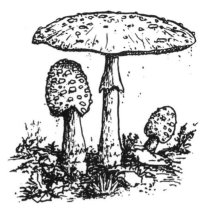

*"Death is the supreme festival
on the road to freedom."*
–Dietrich Bonhoeffer, 1953.

In Europe they once upon a time (and maybe still do) followed their pigs into the forest and gathered the types of mushrooms the pigs were eating. Pigs can sniff a good mushroom before it breaks ground. Unfriendly fungi erupt worldwide, and none ranks as high among the potentially lethal than *Amanita verna* (deadly amanita, death cup, death cap, white amanita, destroying-angel), responsible for approximately 90 percent of all deaths by mushroom.

Look for a chalky white mushroom with a bulbous base, up to nine inches high, four to six inches across the white or yellowish-green to greenish-brown cap when mature, growing the extent of the United States and Canada except on the Pacific Coast. Look for a veil hanging down like a skirt beneath the cap. Look for white or pale gills on the underside of the cap. Look for a mushroom even a pig won't eat.

After a meal of deadly mushroom you'll feel fine for six to 24 hours. Then the complex polypeptides in the 'shroom suddenly produce severe abdominal cramps, profuse puking, watery diarrhea, blurred vision and terrific thirst. Often the symptoms disappear, appear and disappear for periods of time. Don't be misled. The symptoms will usually return one last time with prostration, coma and death, usually within 48 hours. And even if you survive, which sometimes happens, your liver, kidneys and heart will probably never be the same.

Moral: Pick your mushrooms at the grocery store.

The Big Sleep: Deadly Nightshade

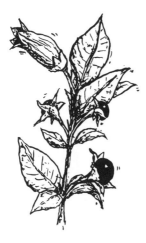

"Beauty is feared, more than death."
—William Carlos Williams,
1948.

Before America figured out it wanted to be a separate and therefore quite distinctive country, *Atropa belladonna*, a member of the widespread and numerous nightshade family (which includes the tomato) came over from Europe for a visit and decided to stay. Bell-shaped and crowded on short branches with many leaves, the reddish, green-yellowish or purple-brownish blooms are still considered of ornamental quality and grown on purpose by some gardeners. "Belladonna" means "beautiful lady." Like many early Americans, these plants escaped the confines of civilization and now grows wild, especially in the East. Although the flowers and leaves, and even the roots, contain poisonous alkaloids, it's the fruit when it ripens to a bright black or purplish-black berry (up to a half-inch across) that can kill, sometimes rather quickly. As few as three berries have been known to end the life of a small child.

As the alkaloids begin to take effect, you'll feel dry in the mouth and have a bit of difficulty swallowing. Your skin will grow warm and look pink; your heartbeat will quicken; your pupils will dilate and you'll have trouble seeing clearly. You may find it difficult to pee. You'll feel a sense of inexplicable excitement as your blood pressure rises and your heartbeat becomes erratic. Your mind will wander into delirium and confusion. As you slip into a coma, a sense of tranquility will pervade, from which comes the name "nightshade." Your respiratory drive will progressively fail... and you'll be dead.

From *Atropa belladonna* come the useful and common drugs atropine and scopolamine. From the beauty of her flowers comes a touch of the sublime. Look and admire the Beautiful Lady... but leave the groping to experts.

Moral: As a wine, deadly nightshade ranks among the last
fluids you'll want in your stemware.

Outwitted by Octopus

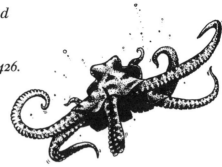

With a bulbous, bag-shaped body (called a mantle) and eight arms, each supplied with two rows of suckers, octopi live worldwide, preferring warmer seas. Octopi are mollusks, relatives of squids (see SQUISHED BY SQUID), cuttlefish and nautiluses, and they hunt by stealth, sneaking up on unsuspecting crabs, crayfish and shellfish, grabbing with their sticky arms and biting with a beak that hides in the heart of the encircling appendages. Octopi stun their victims with a nerve poison and hang out until the squirming prey squirms no more. Without a means to inject their venom, they are relegated to biting and spitting the poison into the wound. Almost all octopi have a venom harmless to humans. Although on rare occasions an unusually large octopus, probably a mentally challenged individual, has been known to leap out of the sea and grab a wading man or woman, death via that means has not occurred, at least not a well-documented death. But don't relax: the colorful and diminutive blue-ringed octopus (*Octopus maculosa*) ranks among the deadliest denizens of the deep blue sea.

Look for blue-ringed octopi off the coasts of eastern and northern Australia, Indonesia and the Philippines. Blue rings circle their arms and blue crescents highlight the purplish-brown bodies of these little octopi. One 10 inches long would be a giant among its peers. When the octopus is irritated or excited, the rings glow an iridescent and lovely peacock blue, which typically happens when an unknowing human picks one of the little creatures up. Their poison is potent, sometimes causing the bitten human to expire in a brief 90 minutes.

The bite is seldom felt, the spit never seen. You may notice a small trickle of blood from the bite site. Within five minutes, maybe a bit more, you'll feel dry in the mouth and have difficulty swallowing as the toxin attacks your nervous system. You will become rapidly and violently ill: vomiting, losing muscular control, collapsing on the beach. Your ability to breathe will become paralyzed, and you'll turn a shade of blue far less appealing than the blue of your killer. You'll pass out before you die.

Moral: Never hug anything with more arms than you.

Offed by Oleander

"A dead man is nothing more than a dead man, and a living man of the slightest pretensions is stronger than the dead man's memory."

—Napoleon I, c. 1804.

Native to the Mediterranean and Asiatic regions of earth, oleander (*Nerium oleander*) has been imported to the United States for its ornamental qualities. A tall shrub, mildly fragrant, the leaves are lance-shaped and leathery, the seed pods long and slender, the seeds hairy and the flowers clustered at the ends of the branches in showy red, white or pink. Its vibrant poisons are the cardiac glycosides oleandrin and nerioside with few equals in the vegetable world. If eaten, a single leaf can eliminate a full-grown adult. Children have succumbed to sucking the nectar from a single flower. Death has taken humans who ate hot dogs impaled and roasted on an oleander branch, or inhaled the smoke from branches thrown into a campfire, or ingested the honey bees made from the juice of oleander flowers. Death has taken horses who ate the leaves, and the plant is called "horse killer" in some parts of the world and "ass killer" in others. Goats, for what it's worth, seem immune.

Almost immediately you'll experience nausea followed by stomach pain and severe vomiting. Watch for bloody diarrhea which should begin in a few hours. You'll feel cold and dizzy, and your heart will slow down and beat irregularly. Drowsiness and unconsciousness will precede a few convulsions and slow paralysis of your ability to breathe. Your death should occur in less than a day.

Moral: Wake up and smell the oleander.

Obliterated by Ostrich

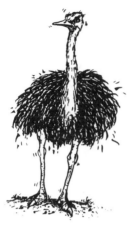

"Even at our birth, death does but stand aside a little. And every day he looks towards us and muses somewhat to himself whether that day or the next he will draw nigh."
–Robert Bolt, 1962.

Not far removed from reptiles, birds are hardly more than warm-blooded lizards with a few other differences such as feathers instead of scales. Birds are creatures of very small brains, which gave rise to the expression "bird-brained" which means, in short, not very smart. Most animals smaller than you will back off when you fight back, but not birds. Even tiny birds will fly at you again and again if they put their tiny minds to it. This is not a big problem unless the bird is not tiny.

The ostrich is the largest bird on earth, a black and white bird, a great flightless bird of Africa that runs faster than humans and reaches heights of nearly eight feet and weights of around 300 pounds. Valued for their feathers and the taste of their meat, ostrich farms are springing up around the world, including the United States.

Ostriches are one of the few birds that will attack a human just because they're having a bad day. And when mating season rolls around, the male ostrich, the cock, is considered by some experts to be among the most volatile and dangerous animals on the surface of the planet.

Ostriches give a terrifically powerful kick with either of their piston-like legs, legs of which the lower half is virtually solid bone ending in two toes (on each leg) with razor-keen toenails. They can only kick forward. Given the right mood and a chance, they'll kick out and down, ripping your guts out and stringing them along the ground as they step in for another kick.

Interesting to note is the fact that ostriches, even the most hysterical cocks, will not kick at or even step on a human lying flat on the ground, although they might peck at you for a while.

Moral: There's much to be said for a low profile.

Partaken Of by Piranha

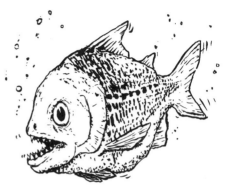

*"We must needs die, and are
as water split on the ground,
which cannot be gathered up
again."*
　　　　　–2 Samuel 14:14.

More than 20 species of piranhas live in the waters of the extensive Amazon Basin, but only four, maybe five of them have ever been known to partake of a human being. Of piranhas, Theodore Roosevelt wrote: "They are the most ferocious fish in the world." Considered the most dangerous, by many experts, but not the largest species, *Serrasalmus natteriri* grows to about 11 inches and travels in immense schools. Their mouths are not that immense, but they are filled with razor sharp teeth that bite with powerful jaws.

Relatively irritable when hungry, piranhas will devour each other if kept enclosed for too long without other food. When shipped, which sometimes happens, piranhas require one container per fish since that's all you'll end up with anyway. When blood spills in piranha-infested water the fish are driven into a veritable feeding frenzy that has reduced many fairly large mammals, including humans, into a pile of bones in remarkably short order, perhaps less than two minutes.

To increase your chances of becoming piranha food, swim in murky waters, which tricks the fish into thinking you're a normal part of their diet, thrash wildly to imitate something in trouble and, for an added guarantee, bleed a little bit.

Moral: Don't feed the fish.

Put Away by Plague

"He that dies pays all debts."

—Shakespeare, The Tempest, 1611.

Between 1347 and 1350, the Black Death, caused by the bacteria *Yersinia pestis*, started in Asia and eventually rubbed out about 25 million Europeans (roughly one-third the population), including nine-tenths of the people of England. Before those devastating years, even in BC days, reports of the ravages of plague were known and feared.

Carried by rodents and passed primarily by the bite of rodent fleas, both rodent and flea are killed by the bacteria, an unusual aspect of this disease. Black rats are especially susceptible, and *Rattus rattus* is blamed for the famous Black Death of Europe. In the United States, deer mice and various voles maintain the bacteria. It is amplified in prairie dogs and ground squirrels. Other suspects include chipmunks, marmots, wood rats, rabbits and hares. States in which plague still exists include New Mexico, Arizona, California, Colorado, Utah, Oregon and Nevada.

Hikers and campers in infected areas may be at risk if they hang out around rodents. Meat-eating pets that eat infected rodents (or get bitten by infected fleas) can acquire plague. Dogs don't get very sick, but cats do. There is only one known case of plague being passed to a human by a dog, but cats can pass the disease to humans by biting them, coughing on them, or carrying their fleas to them. In the wild, coyotes and bobcats are known to have transmitted plague to humans after the critters were dead and the humans were skinning them. Skunks, raccoons and badgers are suspect. Sick people transmit plague readily to other people.

Several forms of plague exist, but the three most common are bubonic, septicemic and pneumonic. (1) Buboes are inflamed, enlarged lymph nodes, and they give bubonic plague its name. After an incubation period of two to six days, you'll usually suffer fever, chills, malaise, muscle aches and headaches. Blackened, bleeding skin sores gave a name to the "Black Death." There's simply no way to look good while you're dying. (2) The septicemic form may appear similar but does not give rise to the ugly buboes. Gastrointestinal pain with nausea, vomiting and diarrhea is common. (3) The pneumonic form results most often from inhaling droplets, say if a sick person coughs on you, but it can develop from bacteria that got into your blood. Coughing often produces blood in the sputum. Death from plague is common and extremely final.

Moral: Flee the flea.

Pulverized by Polar Bear

*"Death takes us piecemeal,
not at a gulp."*
—Seneca, First Century AD.

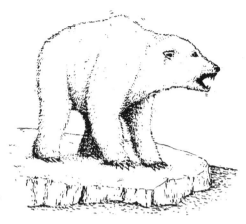

Bears appear worldwide, one of the most diversely distributed mammals on the face of the planet, and they are all relatively similar. But only the polar bear lives entirely off meat. And, being the largest land carnivore on earth (up to 10 feet long, up to 1,600 pounds) and an inhabitant of harsh environments where humans seldom intrude, the polar bear (*Ursus maritimus*) has little fear of humans and no hesitation about feasting on a human if hunger drives them to consume something less appetizing than a fat seal. They prefer seal blubber, skin and organs, and they can sniff out a hunk of blubber from 20 miles away.

These white or yellowish-white bears are perfectly adapted to the typically white landscapes across which they roam. They may cough or roar, but most of their lives are quiet, and quietly they sneak up on their prey for a quick pounce. If necessary, and not their first choice, they can run up to 25 miles per hour to overtake their next meal. They swim well enough to catch sea birds floating on the water. They have even been known to overturn a small boat in order to munch on a less-than-succulent Inuit who happened to be paddling by.

Polar bear attacks on humans follow one of two courses: (1) A hungry bear pulverizes you with one swipe in which your death is usually instantaneous. You are then consumed, organs first. (2) An upset mother bear with a cub or two swipes at you to remind you forcefully to stay away. If you survive the swipe, you may live to see another snowfall.

*Moral: Always travel with someone who runs slower than
you do.*

Poisoned by Puffer Fish

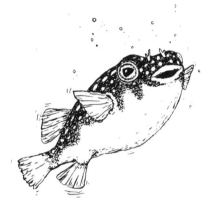

"For the dead there are no more toils."
— *Sophocles, c. 413 BC.*

In Japan, puffer fish (blowfish, globefish, swellfish), precisely prepared, is considered a great delicacy. They call the dish *fugu*. But puffer fish, and their relatives, contain a highly toxic chemical called tetrodotoxin, and improper preparation may give you a case of tetrodotoxin poisoning. Tetrodotoxin is a poison 275 times more potent than cyanide. If your chef toils properly, no organ of the fish touches the soon-to-be-eaten flesh. Death occurs in approximately 60 percent of all cases of puffer fish poisoning, a regular occurrence in less-than-four-star Japanese restaurants.

Over most of the earth, some puffer fish may grow as long as three feet and as heavy as 30 pounds. When threatened they suck water, or air if water isn't available, into an internal bladder "puffing" the fish up two or three times its normal size, a deterrent to predators, the fish hopes. There are about 100 species, warmer seas housing the more poisonous species. If the fish benefits from being poisonous, it is not understood why.

The poison blocks messages from nerves to muscles in humans. In 10 to 45 minutes after dinner, numbness and tingling develop. Vomiting, lightheadedness and a feeling of "impending doom" are commonly reported. Salivation, sweating, chest pain, difficulty swallowing and speaking, convulsions and hypotension may result. Paralysis, difficulty breathing, and a slowed heart rate often lead to death. Survivors often report being paralyzed but totally alert. One wonders if the dead experienced the same phenomena while waiting to pass on.

Moral: A great chef is worth the money.

Quenched by Quicksand

"There is nothing after death,
and death itself is nothing."
—Seneca, First Century AD.

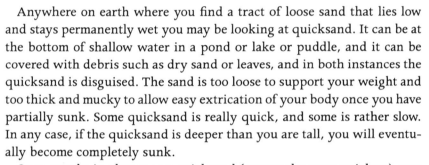

Anywhere on earth where you find a tract of loose sand that lies low and stays permanently wet you may be looking at quicksand. It can be at the bottom of shallow water in a pond or lake or puddle, and it can be covered with debris such as dry sand or leaves, and in both instances the quicksand is disguised. The sand is too loose to support your weight and too thick and mucky to allow easy extrication of your body once you have partially sunk. Some quicksand is really quick, and some is rather slow. In any case, if the quicksand is deeper than you are tall, you will eventually become completely sunk.

Once caught in almost any quicksand (except the very quickest), you can throw yourself flat on your back and float and gently swim to the edge and crawl out. Thrashing around wildly, however, increases substantially your rate of sinking. After your head goes under, you'll hold your breath as long as you can, then you'll inhale a bunch of sand and lose consciousness and, in a few minutes, your brain will shut down totally. If you do not sink in over your head, you'll have to stand around until you die of starvation. Either way, you have saved the cost of a gravesite.

Moral: Never get into anything over your head.

Ravaged by Rabies

"Man is the only animal that contemplates death, and also the only animal that shows any sign of doubt of its finality."

—William Ernest Hocking, 1957.

Around 2000 BC in Mesopotamia, physicians first described the horror of dying from rabies. The agonizing difficulty in swallowing, the pain sometimes caused by the mere sight of water, produced the common name of hydrophobia (fear of water). Estimates place the annual number of human rabies deaths worldwide somewhere between 50,000 and 100,000.

Shaped like an ultramicroscopic bullet, the virus, carried in the saliva of infected animals, attaches itself to peripheral nerves at the bite site and moves slowly but with great determination along nerves toward the brain. Since rabies causes no reaction until it reaches the central nervous system, you don't know you're infected until it's too late. Once replication of the virus starts in the brain, nasty deaths have invariably resulted. Before death, after multiplying, the virus moves back out along nerves, congregating in different body parts including skin, corneas, and in salivary glands at which time you, too, can pass the virus.

Only 33 documented cases of rabies have been reported in the United States since 1977. And at least 12 of the dead people acquired the virus on trips to foreign lands. Often thought of as a disease of carnivores, any mammal can theoretically have rabies, and cows are the most common domestic animal to carry the disease. Despite the publicity mad dogs have received, rabid cats outnumber rabid dogs. The last two decades have shown a steady increase in the number of wild animals having the virus: raccoons, skunks and bats are most dangerous, followed by foxes and coyotes. Foxes are the leading source of rabies in Europe, mongooses in Puerto Rico, dogs in Africa, South America and most of Asia, wolves and jackals in India and Israel.

Early symptoms of rabies are too general to cause concern: fatigue, headache, irritability, depression, nausea, fever, stomach pain. Sounds like another day at the office. There is only one way to know for sure if you have the disease. You die! But first: wild hallucinations, including episodes of unexplainable terror, extremely painful difficulty swallowing to the point where you refuse all liquids and drool constantly, frequent muscle spasms especially in the face and neck, and, toward the end, complete disorientation and a raging fever.

Moral: Don't feed the mouth that bites.

Ripped by Rattlesnake

*"Death's dark way must
needs be trodden once,
however we pause."*
        –Horace, c. 15 BC.

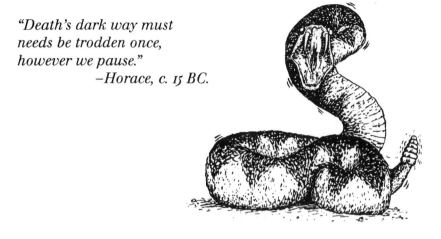

Living somewhere on earth today are approximately 2,700 kinds of snakes. Roughly 412 species are venomous enough to cause serious complications in the life of a human. In the United States, members of two families of snakes have bites that could prove lethal: the Elapidae (see CORRALLED BY CORAL SNAKE) and the Crotalidae, the pit vipers, whose membership includes the rattlesnakes. Not all the Crotalidae have rattles (see MASSACRED BY MOCCASIN), but all rattlesnakes have rattles. Although there is room for argument among the experts, there seem to be about 30 species and subspecies of rattlesnakes rattling around in the United States. In addition to rattles, they all have a specialized venom injection system that works extremely well. It works like this: Venom is manufactured and stored in glands near the roots of two long, sharp, curved, hinged fangs. When the snake strikes, the mouth opens with the upper jaw almost 180 degrees from the lower jaw. The fangs spring 90 degrees down from the upper jaw and penetrate their victim. Venom is immediately squirted down the hollow fangs and out a small orifice slightly above the point and in the front of the fang.

Diamondback rattlesnakes, the Western and slightly larger Eastern, cause most of the 10 to 15 deaths per year via snake in the United States. Although the snake may not envenomate with every bite, the venom causes immediate and intense pain, and rapid swelling near the wound. In small creatures, say a mouse, the venom is carried through the bloodstream and starts to dissolve the victim for easier digestion after being swallowed whole. In you the same process starts but you won't totally dissolve. Just some of you dissolves, especially near where you got bit. Your red blood cells are broken down so they can no longer carry oxygen, and if enough of them are broken down, internal bleeding erupts, organs start to fail, cardiovascular shock rears its ugly head, you feel terrible and you bite the dust.

Since rattlesnakes bite 7,000 to 8,000 humans in the United States every year, the chance that you'll be one to die is relatively small. But if life has got you down, there's always a chance. Running around and screaming after being bitten increases your chances.

Moral: *There's a lot to be said for staying calm and watching your step.*

Ruined by Recluse

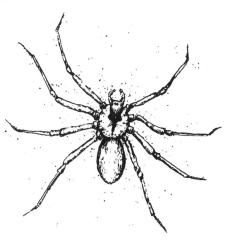

*"Pain lays not its touch upon
a corpse."*
        —Aeschylus, c. 456 BC.

Brown spiders or brown recluses
(*Loxosceles reclusa*), sometimes
called fiddlebacks, are faun to dark
brown in color, grow to an inch or
slightly more across, have long legs
and a dark violin-shape on their topsides with the neck of the violin reaching toward their rear end. They're common in the Southern States, up the Mississippi Valley and are spreading around the United States. A rather cosmopolitan creature, they are at home in homes: under houses, beneath beds, in the backs of closets, in the arms and legs of old clothes you haven't worn for a year or so. But, if you're interested in being bitten by one, rest assured they haunt the outdoors as well, preferring to hide out in piles of brush, old rodent nests and under logs. Being independent of webs, they hunt at night, stalking their prey. That's when they bite humans. Not because they think you're food, but because you bump into them with your bare feet, roll over on them while they're crossing your sleeping body or stick your hand into where they're hiding.

Stinging pain usually soon follows a recluse bite, but sometimes bitees report no initial pain. Stinging will subside after six to eight hours, to be replaced by an ache and itching that starts around the bite site, which turns red surrounded by white. Fever, chills, weakness, nausea and vomiting may ruin a day or two. Before too awful long a bubble forms, filled with blood or clear fluid. Then a scab forms. Then the scab falls off, leaving a nasty wound that looks sort of like a third degree burn. It is extremely difficult to get this wound to heal.

Death could occur in a couple of ways. One, infection from the wound could spread throughout your body. Two, the venom could, though only rarely, ruin your kidneys. Either way you would fall into a very small category of Causes of Death. How interesting!

Moral: Never fiddle around with dangerous things.

Rubbed Out by Red Tide

"This fell sergeant, Death, is strict in his arrest."
—Shakespeare, Hamlet, 1600.

As sea currents bring in denser, cooler wedges of water from offshore, seeds of dinoflagellates are stirred up from their rest on the sea floor. These micro-algae are then exposed to enough sunlight and warm surface temperatures to bloom. They live through a single reproductive cycle and drop new seeds to the bed of the ocean to await another shift in the restless sea. These unicellular plankton are the foundation of the food chain, ranking second in abundance only to diatoms.

Inside the cell of a limited number of dinoflagellates, called *Alexandrium catenella*, toxins are produced. The most common toxin encountered in the United States is saxitoxin. It is odorless and colorless and tasteless. If the concentration of these *A. catenella* dinoflagellates is high enough, they color the ocean: red tide. But a red tide does not have to occur for the dinoflagellates to be present in toxic numbers.

Many birds and fish are killed by eating the red blooms, but many shellfish (oysters, clams, mussels, scallops) store the toxins in their gills and digestive organs while suffering no ill effect. If you eat a "bad" shellfish, raw or cooked, the result could be paralytic shellfish poisoning. Shortly after consumption tingling starts in your lips and mouth. You won't have to wait long for abdominal cramping, nausea, vomiting, diarrhea, lightheadedness, headache, difficulty with your vision, incoherence and loss of coordination due to a creeping paralysis. If the paralysis creeps far enough, you'll lose the ability to breathe and retire forever to that oyster bed in the sky.

Moral: Clam up before it's too late.

Wrecked by Rhinoceros

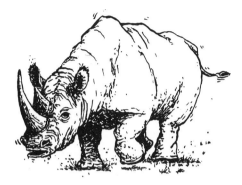

"The last act is tragic, however happy all the rest of the play is; at the last a little earth is thrown upon our head, and that is the end for ever."
        –Pascal, 1670.

Descended from the largest land mammals ever to roam the earth, a creature at least 18 feet at the shoulder, rhinoceroses are kin to horses but have grown very thick hides and a horn or two on their noses. Once numbered in the hundreds of thousands, currently the world enjoys fewer rhinos than American bison. Their name comes from the Greek word *rhinokeros*, "nose horn," and there are five species on today's earth: Indian rhinos, Javan rhinos, Sumatran or "hairy" rhinos, white rhinos and black rhinos. All are nearsighted and short-tempered, keen of smell and keen on trampling anything that lies in their path when they suddenly erupt into high speed charges. Africa's black rhino is rated the greatest opportunity for death.

The reaction of rhinos to an unusual sound (the click of a camera, the rustle of grass) or smell (you) is to charge over at full speed to find out what's going on. They have been known to charge full speed, about 35 miles per hour, into cars, buses, even trains. A myth surrounding a rhino's charge is that you can wait until the last moment and quickly side step. Unless you're Tarzan, it won't work! A rhino in full charge can turn on a dime and give five cents change, and they have the nasty habit of hooking right and left with their horns when they get within striking range. The result is you are often caught on the horn and tossed 12 feet or so into the air. If the rhino misses with the horn, it will probably plow you underground beneath its thundering feet. Either way, or both ways at once, you tend to be quite dead and messy by the time a rhinoceros figures out you are no particular threat.

Moral: Stay away from horny neighbors.

Stung by Scorpion

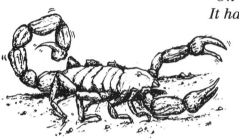

"Oh Death where is thy sting?
It has none. But life has."
—Mark Twain, 1935.

Nothing much, or perhaps nothing at all, has changed for scorpions in the last 400 million years or so, give or take a few millennia, except there are far more feet trying to stomp them to death. Arachnids, they still scuttle rapidly on eight legs, relatives of the spider, with lobster-like pincers to grab and rend their prey and a five-segmented "tail" which is actually the end of their abdomen. A single sharp stinger at the end of the tummy has two orifices of extremely small size fed by two relatively large venom glands. They are nocturnal and solitary, aggressive and sometimes deadly to humans.

Found almost everywhere, scorpions are most common in the tropics and in other warm climates. Of the approximately 650 species of scorpions worldwide, about 40 species are known to scuttle in the United States. Of those 40 only the attractively slim and sculpted and pale yellowish *Centruroides*, found in the Southwest, regularly ends human life, usually in a child. Death by scorpion is far more common in India, where species such as the dreaded and dangerous and darkly black *Palamneus* lurks in every other nook and cranny.

They will sneak into your tent or sleeping bag, hide in your clothes and boots and under rocks, bark and leaves. When the abdomen curls up, the scorpion is ready to sting with the speed of greased lightning. The result is almost instant pain from the richly neurotoxic poison which attacks the victim's nerves.

If you know you're in scorpion country, look before you put your hands or feet into dark places, shake out your clothing and boots every morning, and your sleeping bag every night. Otherwise, as the toxin takes effect from a deadly scorpion, the localized burning pain may spread to your abdomen, and you'll curl up in sheer torture. With cold and clammy skin, you will shiver and shake, sweat profusely and vomit several violent times. You will have increasing difficulty breathing as you slip closer and closer to respiratory failure. finally, 12 to 15 agonizing hours later, with frothy fluid bubbling from your nose and mouth, you will slough off this mortal shell.

Moral: A tail may be more than a tale.

Screwed by Screwworm Fly

"Why, do you not know, then, that the origin of all human evils, and of baseness, and cowardice, is not death, but rather the fear of death?"

—Epictetus, Second Century BC.

Many species of flies have the repugnant habit of laying their eggs in dead meat. The eggs hatch into maggots, which tenderize the dead meat with their excrement so they can eat it and eventually become adult flies. The screwworm fly (*Callitroga americana* in the Americas, *Chrysomya bessiana* in Africa and Asia), blue-green to purplish-black in color, has an even nastier habit.

Female screwworm flies lay their eggs in the wounds of living meat. Any wound will do, even a small scratch. If given free reign, she will lay between 500 and 3,000 eggs over a three to five day period. The eggs hatch in about 24 hours, and the maggots, each about a half inch at maturity, each looking somewhat like a small screw, eat their way with surprising rapidity into the living animal. In screwworm fly areas, deaths among cows and sheep can be astounding, death taking place when the maggots eat into the brain or lungs, which can take from a few days to a week.

It will probably all start for you while you're asleep. The screwworm fly lays her eggs in, say, where you scratched a mosquito bite. Before you know it, a substantial part of your body has been eaten away. Your death will be unlikely via screwworm fly unless for some reason you decide to let the maggots keep screwing around with you. Or someone tied you to a tree in a fly-infested cow pasture.

Moral: A swat in time saves lives.

Snuffed by Scuba

"Man imagines that it is death he fears; but what he fears is the unforeseen, the explosion."

—Saint-Exupery, 1942.

Scuba has been used as a stand-alone word for so long many humans have forgotten that it is an acronym for *self-contained underwater breathing apparatus*, originally an invention of Jacques Cousteau. Scuba divers breathe air highly compressed into a tank. The air is fed to the diver through a regulator that regulates the pressure of the air being inhaled. As the diver descends under water, air pressure increases dramatically, doubling at 33 feet, but the pressure of inhaled air from the tank remains the same. Everything works fine as long as the diver does not stay down too long, does not come up too fast and remembers to keep breathing.

A diver who stays down too long or comes up too fast often has the nitrogen in the air being breathed form bubbles inside his or her body. The bubbles put pressure on tissues and cause pain. This is called "the bends" because bending (flexing) joints increases the pain. Death is rare, but permanent paralysis is not exceedingly rare.

If you are a diver who forgets to keep breathing, who holds his or her breath, you can have a serious problem if you ascend at the same time. The air inside your chest starts to increase in size as the ambient air pressure decreases on ascent. The increase in the space air takes up in your chest can cause injury from a depth as shallow as four feet. Suddenly your chest will explode. Not your chest, exactly, but parts of your lungs pop, making it very difficult to breath. Air bubbles can enter your bloodstream through the rips, and enter your brain, causing a stroke-like death within minutes.

Moral: Never hold your breath underwater... when you're scuba diving.

Silenced by Sea Snake

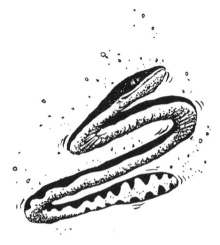

"Sunset and evening star,
and one clear call for me!
And may there be no
moaning of the bar, when I
put out to sea."
—Alfred Lord Tennyson, 1889.

Sea snakes, each and every one of the approximately 50 species, are venomous. Members of the family Hydrophiidae, they live almost exclusively in the western Pacific and Indian Oceans. One exception is the Yellow-bellied sea snake whose range includes the entire Pacific Ocean to the coast of Mexico and south. Four to six feet in average length, some species may reach 10 feet or more. Air breathers, they must return to the surface regularly in order to survive. Living their lives in a liquid medium, however, has produced unique adaptations in the snake world. Slender in the front half, they flatten toward the rear into a paddlelike tail that allows them to swim with great finesse and to strike with agility by "springing" off their tails. Varying in toxicity, at least one species has venom rated as 50 times more potent than a King cobra. Their fangs are like a cobra, short and fixed, hollow and relatively small. Packing a virulent nerve toxin, sea snakes are among the most poisonous of creatures.

They prefer to bite and consume small fish, but they bite humans, too, usually when they are accidentally handled or stepped on in shallow water. Most victims report little pain, and most sea snake venom is relatively slow acting, although symptoms may appear is some cases within minutes. Within hours, surely, you'll feel growing anxiety, muscle stiffness and muscle aches. The pain grows. Spastic paralysis follows. Nausea and vomiting typically complicate your remaining hours, which are often further characterized by restlessness, loss of bowel control and deep unhappiness. Just before your ability to breathe fails, you'll have difficulty seeing. But, heck, you'll have little interest in looking at anything by that time.

Moral: See snake, sea snake, never touch a snake.

Savaged by Seal

"The most rational cure after all for the inordinate fear of death is to set a just value on life."

—William Hazlitt, 1821.

Of the 47 kinds of pinnipeds (see WASTED BY WALRUS) that swim the earth's water with a mermaid-like tail, none ranks as more fierce of aspect when confronted with a human than the leopard seal (*Hydrurga leptonyx*). A resident of difficult-to-access areas of the Antarctic and sub-Antarctic, leopard seal males grow to 10 feet and 600-plus pounds while the females may reach 12 feet and 1,000 pounds. Like all seals, leopard seals are naturally inquisitive, but, for the most part, would rather have nothing at all to do with humans. Birds, especially penguins, top the list of preferred foods, but hard times will send them to the fish market, and they are not opposed to hunting down and eating other species of seals, some of which are two or three times human size. Streamlined with a strong and flexible neck, agile and mighty swift in the water, they are rather awkward when they haul out on land or ice, and an average man or woman should be able to outrun an outraged leopard seal. When they are bothered, most notably when the males have formed a harem for breeding or they are being attacked by human hunters for their hide, they sneer and open their large mouths, baring their large teeth but remaining remarkably quiet.

Leopard seals lunge and bite with long, sharp teeth that curve inward. They don't chew. They grip with their powerful jaw muscles and shake their heads until something small enough to swallow whole rips off their prey. Not the smallest shred of evidence exists indicating leopard seals eat human meat. But, nonetheless, they are most definitely capable of being pressed hard enough to kill you.

Moral: The unwise seal their own doom.

Swallowed by Sperm Whale

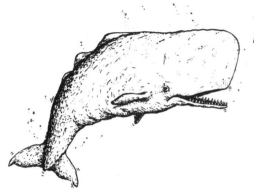

*"Death is one moment, and
life is so many of them."*
— *Tennessee Williams, 1963.*

Whales, gentle giants of the sea, have little wish to cross paths with humans, largely due to the fact that humans have hunted and killed them for hundreds of years. Yet, even when threatened, whales rarely cause harm to humans, and those rare times are often by accident. Sperm whales (*Physeter catodon*), growing to 60 feet in length, occasionally produce what some experts refer to as a "rogue male," an individual documented to batter ships and break and drown seamen. And, even less often, to swallow humans.

In February of 1891, the whaling ship *Star of the East* harpooned a sperm whale in the South Atlantic, east of the Falkland Islands. Young James Bartley, on his apprentice voyage, was thrown from the longboat when the maddened whale beat the sea to a froth. He disappeared. Whale's blood had attracted a congregation of sharks, and Bartley was given up as shark food.

The whale died and was tied to the side of the ship and slowly butchered. When the whale's stomach was thrown aboard, it jumped as if alive. James Bartley was removed from the stomach, still breathing, bleached white and hairless, almost blind. Approximately 15 hours had elapsed since the young man's disappearance. He lived long enough to return to England and tell his tale of falling into the whale's mouth, of screaming as he washed over the rows of tiny sharp teeth, of sliding down a long slimy tube, of blissful oblivion in the belly of the great mammal.

Moral: Some things are easier to swallow than others.

Felled by
Rocky Mountain Spotted Fever

"Life is strewn with so many dangers, and can be the source of so many misfortunes, that death is not the greatest of them."
                                        —Napolean I, c. 1804.

Transmitted by the bite of ticks, Rocky Mountain spotted fever is not limited to the Rocky Mountains and, in fact, was first recognized in the northwestern United States about 200 years ago and now has been identified all over the Western Hemisphere. Neither is it a fever with spots. It is a disease which gives *you* a spotty rash and a high fever. The cause is a bacteria that lives well inside of ticks, especially wood ticks and American dog ticks, a bacteria (*Rickettsia rickettsii*) of the family Rickettsiaceae, a bacteria that may live well inside of you. The ticks feed on any warm-blooded mammal. If the mammal has the bacteria, ticks pick it up and pass it to you should they find your warm blood available at meal time.

The incubation period, the time from the tick bite until you know you're sick, can range from two to 14 days. Along with the sudden onset of fever, chills, headache and muscle aches, you will develop a rash that spreads over your entire body, including the palms of your hands and the soles of your feet. You may also have stomach pain, vomiting, diarrhea and confusion about what's going on. You have a fairly OK chance of surviving, but the bacteria invade the walls of your blood vessels, primarily your arteries and arterioles, and your heart muscle and can collapse your vasculature within as little as six days of the tick bite. Untreated, about three out of ten humans die from Rocky Mountain spotted fever.

Removal of the imbedded tick before it feeds can prevent the disease (see LICKED BY LYME DISEASE). When you check for ticks remember they prefer to feed on the warm, dark, moist, embarrassing areas of your body.

Moral: You can learn who your real friends are at tick check time.

Squished by Squid

"The descent to Hades is
much the same from
whatever place we start."
–Anaxagoras, Sixth Century BC.

If there be monsters in the sea, then they are probably giant squids, *Architeuthis*, who live way down deep, whose length remains even today a source of debate with estimates ranging from a mere 60 feet to a whopping 300 feet. To the old Norse they were called kraken. To fishermen before the birth of Christ they were feared as Godless destroyers who rose to the surface after dark to drag down boats straggling in late toward shore. Frank W. Lane in his *Kingdom of the Octopus* says squid "are the most ferocious of all invertebrates."

In addition to their eight arms, squid have two long tentacles which they shoot out with amazing speed to capture and haul in prey to their beaks for shredding and consuming. Distributed worldwide, they might rise to any surface of any ocean.

The passenger steamer *Strathowen*, bound from Columbo to Madras, witnessed on 31 July 1874 an attack on the *Pearl*, 150 tons of schooner: "Someone on the schooner fired a rifle at the (large brownish mass) and it began to move toward the schooner and squeezed on board between the fore and mainmast, pulling the vessel over and sinking it. Its body was as thick as the schooner and about half as long, with a train that appeared to be 100 feet long." The *Strathowen* picked up the survivors. The creature's tentacles "which were as thick as a barrel" crushed the other members of the crew. You can't say that about very many dead humans.

Moral: Leave well enough alone.

Stunned by Stonefish

"Death is the supple Suitor
that wins at last..."
—Emily Dickinson, c. 1878.

Inhabiting the sea floor in tropical waters, and occasionally in temperate waters, scorpionfish, family Scorpaenidae, sting with sharp spines that stick out their backs like a row of poison-tipped nails. Some of the family members are lovely and graceful (lionfish, firefish) and carry a painful venom that produces voracious pain. Some of these fish are exceedingly unattractive, lumps of flesh that resemble a part of the coral reef they call home more than a finned saltwater denizen. None of them are less appealing or more dangerous than the stonefish (genus *Synanceja*) who provides not only pain but also an opportunity to die, whose poison is rated as an equal to cobra venom.

If you inadvertently step on a stonefish, the most common way to make contact, one of the spines can easily puncture through sneakers or flippers, and pressure on the spine forces the venom up two paired ducts into your foot (or hand if you happen to reach for a stonefish). If provoked, stonefish typically attack. Pain is immediate and immeasurably intense, but that's only the beginning. In 60 to 90 minutes the pain will peak and stay peaked for six to 12 hours, pain cruel enough to drive the wimpy insane. Screaming is very common. Death in humans is fairly rare but often preferred by victims since it usually drops you in six to eight hours so you don't have to suffer so much. If you live you'll have disconcerting stuff to look forward to in addition to the pain: headache, rash, nausea, vomiting, diarrhea, stomach pain, heavy sweating, arm and leg paralysis, fever, delirium and seizures, to name a few of the more well known effects.

Moral: You can learn things even from what appears to be a stone.

Terrified by Taipan

"Even Rome cannot grant us a dispensation from death."
                                              −Moliere, 1665.

Australia houses the world's greatest variety of snakes known collectively as elapids (family Elapidae) with at least 85 named kinds of these rather insolent, venomous reptiles whose fangs are short and fixed in their upper jaws. Elapids, which include the cobras, cause more human deaths than any other snake family, and one Australian family member is worthy of special note.

If you were zipped into your dome tent with any snake, which one would give you the least chance of survival? When asked a similar question, a panel of experts unanimously voted the King cobra as "most dangerous" (see CLOBBERED BY COBRA). Running second, but not far behind, was Australia's taipan (*Oxyuranus scutellatus*), growing to lengths of over 10 feet, a coastal snake of typically light and unremarkable color. Scarce and rarely seen, quick to run when threatened, taipans counter-attack when you try to pick one up. They suddenly turn ferocious, biting savagely and displaying a definite unwillingness to let go. Some victims, indeed, report having great difficulty removing the snake.

The neurotoxic venom will tend to cause a creeping paralysis that first affects your ability to speak, see, swallow and hold your eyes open. Your arms and legs will begin to weaken. If you survive, which sometimes happens, you'll probably have a lot of trouble healing the rotting muscles where the taipan bit. If you die, it will be preceded by a period of increasing difficulty breathing until you no longer can. Some humans have lived through the difficult breathing stage only to die later when their kidneys failed.

Moral: Never pick up what you may not be able to put down.

Trapped by Tetanus

"Every tiny part of us cries out against the idea of dying, and hopes to live forever."

—Ugo Betti, 1949.

Spores of hardy *Clostridium tetani* rank among the world's most common bacterial inhabitants of soil and vegetation. Approximately one out of every 10 humans carries the bacteria in their intestinal tracts. When they get into an anaerobic environment, say trapped in the bottom of a dirty wound, the spores germinate and release a toxin. This toxin, tetanospasmin, causes the disease tetanus.

The incubation period may run from one to 55 days, but symptoms tend to show up within two weeks. Tetanospasmin spreads throughout your nervous system, where it interferes with the production of inhibitory neurotransmitters, which means you start having violent muscular spasms. Rigidity of your jaw muscles (called trismus or "lockjaw") with difficulty swallowing will usually be your first complaints. Expect signs of sympathetic nervous system involvement: rapid heart rate, sweating, a rise in blood pressure. Seizures are common. Breathing may become difficult and respiratory failure will probably be the immediate cause of your death.

Recognized since the days of the medically oriented Greeks, mortality rates for tetanus, even today, approach 40 percent in adults and 90 percent in children. That's why even tiny babies are vaccinated against the disease.

Moral: Don't leave home without being up-to-date against tetanus.

Slain by Siberian Tiger

"Men are convinced of your arguments, your sincerity, and the seriousness of your efforts only by your death."

—Albert Camus, 1956.

Approximately 40 different wild cats inhabit the earth today, none growing larger than the great Siberian tiger, which reaches 12 feet in length and 400 to 650 pounds in weight. The greatest of the great tipped the scales at 850 pounds. With a base color of bright reddish-orange to white and bold black stripes, this tiger grows exceptionally long fur to protect it from the intense winters of its range, the vast and frigid Siberian territory. Sometimes covering an area as large as 4,000 square miles, spending most of their time alone and hunting, Siberian tigers have been documented to wander over 600 miles in search of food which, when given a choice, will be deer or wild pig. Their immense strength allows them to drag loads that would tax the might of a dozen strong men at once. They need to average about 20 pounds of meat per day to survive, and think nothing of polishing off 100 pounds at one meal. They rarely kill humans, possibly because there are less than 100 that have so far escaped the ravages of humans.

The Siberian tiger is a stalker, creeping to within 30 to 80 feet before charging an intended victim. Should it happen to be you, you will be grabbed by the neck while the tiger's feet remain firmly planted on the ground. If you survive the initial attack, the tiger will hold on very firmly, squeezing your neck until you suffocate. Your body will be dragged to a comfortable spot, usually near water, where the cat feeds until satiated. What remains of you will be buried while the tiger takes a break and typically falls asleep. Later you'll be dug up and finished off. Not fun, but definitely interesting.

Moral: When in Siberia, avoid smelling of pig and saying things like "Here, kitty, kitty, kitty."

Torn Apart by Tiger Shark

"We dread life's termination as the close, not of enjoyment, but of hope."

—William Hazlitt, 1817.

Sharks appeared before dinosaurs and have managed to thrive for about 350 million years. They circle the globe, preferring tropical and subtropical seas but being well documented to swim north to the Arctic. They have been caught as deep as 9,000 feet, and probably live even deeper. Without bones, they are made of stout and flexible cartilage, covered by incredibly rough skin, and teeth, lots of teeth, teeth that are soon replaced should one fall out, sharp teeth powered by monstrous jaw muscles. With an almost supernatural ability to sense prey, sharks can detect blood in water at no more than one part per million. Small of brain, large and voracious of appetite, sharks are killing "devices," and humans, although not a favored food of sharks, are by no means excepted.

Tiger sharks (*Galeocerdo cuvieri*) develop faded darker gray vertical stripes on their lighter gray bodies and grow to 14 feet, the largest shark on Pacific reefs, often seen from South Carolina south and in the Bahamas, a shark easily cataloged as one of the species most dangerous to humans. Ravenous hunger and poor eyesight have sent them after humans as food numerous times. Ravenous hunger and poor eyesight, in fact, have sent them after metal, wood, leather and plastic, giving tiger sharks the nickname of "garbage cans of the sea." They seem to prefer birds and turtles for food, but these sharks will consume anything the sea provides, more often feeding at night in shallow waters.

Keenly serrated, the teeth of a tiger shark tend to raggedly tear off parts of you after the shark bites and as it shakes its head. Your blood loss will be immediate and immense. After swallowing, the shark will return for another bite. On a happier note, there probably won't be enough time for you to feel pain. Soon a red smear delicately shading the water will be all that's left of you.

Moral: In the water at day, usually OK; in the water at night, tiger shark's delight.

Twisted by Tornado

"The worst evil of all is to leave the ranks of the living before one dies."

—Seneca, First Century AD.

Thunderstorms and hailstorms are related to tornadoes and classified as "locally severe storms." Local storms routinely display high winds, but tornadoes go a twist further, spiraling inward and upward in a vortex that can be of incredible power. The bottom of the vortex (the funnel) can be several yards to several hundred yards wide and reach up from several yards to more than mile high with the roar of a closely passing jet. The top of the vortex consists primarily of water droplets and the bottom of dirt and dust and anything else the wind sucks up. Tornadoes occur most often and most devastatingly in the United States, and are most likely in spring and summer. Tornadoes have shredded strips of countryside a mile wide and more than 100 miles long. They have picked up loaded freight cars from trains and thrown them through office buildings. They have ripped houses into tiny pieces. They have driven straws through trees. They have taken a little girl and her dog from Kansas to Oz.

Your greatest opportunity to die in a tornado comes when you stand outside exposing yourself to whatever the storm has turned into a speeding missile: boards, bricks, limbs of trees, cows, small imported cars. You can also be picked up and turned into a speeding missile yourself, your demise coming shortly after you are slammed into the ground or anything else standing in your flight path.

Moral: Adding a new twist to our life can be dangerous.

Tricked by Trichinosis

"All human things are subject to decay, and when fate sum-mons, monarchs must obey."

–John Dryden, 1682.

Encysted in skeletal muscle, the larvae of the parasitic worm *Trichinella spiralis* are eaten by some hungry meat eater. In the small intestine, the worms mature and mate within a few days, usually within 48 hours. Fe-male worms deposit larvae in nearby mucosal tissue. Larvae enter the circulatory system of the animal and invade skeletal muscle. Within three weeks, the larvae are encysted and ready to be infectiously passed should anything eat the muscle of the animal that ate the muscle of the animal that had encysted larvae.

Although all carnivorous or omnivorous mammals may have trichinosis, consumption of raw or undercooked pork accounts for the vast majority of the disease in humans. Rodents are often infected, but mice and rats seldom grace a human palate. Bears, raccoons, opossums, seals, walruses, peccaries and wild swine are common hosts, and sometimes are eaten by humans.

Trichinosis produces gastrointestinal symptoms during the first week after ingestion of infected meat: pain, nausea, vomiting, variable diar-rhea. The severity of the symptoms depends on the number of larvae eaten. During the second week, as the larvae migrate around your body, capillary damage occurs, commonly producing facial edema, and maybe producing hemorrhages in nail beds and your conjunctiva. Migrating lar-vae can invade the pulmonary system, causing a cough and chest pain, or the heart muscle, causing carditis and a chance at patient death. Gas-trointestinal symptoms may remain for four to six weeks, until the worms are all excreted. As the larvae encyst in muscle tissue, significant muscle aches and stiffness often result. Between six and 18 months after inges-tion, the larvae die and become calcified. This period is usually asymptomatic, and if you made it this far, you'll have to wait for another way to die.

Moral: Pigs can't swim and pigs can't fly, but pigs can
sometimes make you die.

Tucked In by Tsetse Fly

"There is no God found stronger than death; and death is a sleep."

—Algernon Charles Swinburne, 1866.

Although fossil evidence indicates they once buzzed around the prehistoric skies of North America, the brownish tsetse fly (family Glossinidae) now lives only in tropical Africa. They feed in daylight and they feed on blood and human blood is totally satisfying to the hungry fly. When driven by hunger, tsetse flies swarm viciously, bite through heavy clothing and rhino hide and even attack the closed windows of vehicles. The bite is briefly painful and itchy.

Born free of disease organisms, baby fly larvae feed off glands in mom for a while, then burrow into the ground to reappear 30 to 40 days later as a full blown fly. They leave the ground immediately in search of blood, and drink up to three times their weight at a feeding. If the animal they drink from is infected with microscopic trypanosomes, which is often the case, the fly now carries these disease-causing organisms.

If you are bitten by a trypanosome-bearing tsetse, the single-celled parasites enter your bloodstream. They multiply rapidly and start eating your own body's glucose. Bad things will start with a headache and fever and progress to increasing lethargy. You'll stumble your way through a period of anemia, seizures and delirium before you slip into a coma during which the "tryps" slowly take over. To the outside world you appear deeply asleep for a period of a few weeks to, perhaps, a few years. Death from sleeping sickness (trypanosomiasis) is brought to you by the thirst of the tsetse fly.

Moral: Walk softly and carry a big fly swatter.

Tswept Away by Tsunami

"Life and death appear more certainly ours than whatsoever else; and yet hardly can that be called ours, which comes without our knowledge, and goes without it."
—Walter Savage Landor, c. 1824.

A word in Japanese than means "harbor wave," a tsunami is often called a tidal wave, but these mightily destructive rushes of sea water have nothing at all to do with tides. They are the result, most often, of the shifting of geologic faults in the floor of the sea. They can also be caused by huge underwater or land-into-water landslides and underwater volcanic eruptions. Not a single wave, tsunamis are series of waves, sometimes more than 10. Unlike everyday waves which may reach speeds of 60 miles per hour, tsunamis have been clocked at nearly 500 miles per hour. While normal waves roll along about 300 yards or so apart, the successive crests of tsunamis may be as much as 90 *miles* apart.

Although a tsunami passing under a ship at sea may go almost unnoticed, the waves slow and increase in height as they near the shore. The first sign of impending danger is typically a sudden rush of water *away* from shore, leaving a long stretch of sea floor exposed and fish flopping helplessly on the bared bottom. Then the mad rush of water rolls toward land, maybe as a high wall and maybe not. Failing to stop where the sea usually stops, the tsunami keeps on coming inland. The record tsunami rushed 1740 feet past the high water mark in Lituya Bay, AK.

You don't have to be outdoors to be killed by a tsunami, but it helps. Waves can get you going and coming. The inland rush of water may be great enough to raze everything in its path and tumble you along until you have drowned. But if it misses on the first try, the wild withdrawal of a tsunami back into the sea irresistably sucks everything with it.

Moral: Never camp less than 1740 feet from the ocean.

Tortured by Tularemia

"Hardest of deaths to a mortal is the death he sees ahead."
—Bacchylides, Fifth Century BC.

Since 1967, less than 200 cases per year have been diagnosed in the United States. The Japanese physician Soken first spotted the disease in people who got sick from eating "bad" rabbit meat in the year 1837. In 1912 the disease was isolated in rodents in Tulare County, California, and thus the sickness, caused by coccobacillus *Francisella tularensis*, acquired its common name of tularemia.

Though certainly once a disease associated with unhealthy contact with rabbits, ticks are now, by far, considered the prime transmission mode for the bacteria. Although many species of ticks have been incriminated, dog ticks and lone star ticks rank as the most common reservoirs. Since the infecting organisms have not been found in tick saliva, it is thought they are carried in tick feces. Think about that! Rabbits still qualify as the second most common vector, but you must handle infected tissue, as you might do by skinning and eviscerating the little bunny. You could pick the disease up in water or soil, too, by direct contact, ingestion or breathing in contaminated dust or water particles.

Most cases appear as a sudden onset of high fever and headache. About 80 percent of tularemia cases appear in an ulceroglandular form: red bumps harden and ulcerate, usually on the lower extremities where ticks bit, or on the hands from handling infected tissues. Ulcers are typically painful and tender. Enlarged tender lymph nodes are common. The second most common form of tularemia, the typhoidal form, causes fever, chills and debility. Weight loss may be significant. Lymph node enlargement is less. Pneumonia is a relatively common complication of tularemia. If you can work up a serious pneumonia, you can increase your chances of dying from five percent to 30 percent.

Moral: It may not be "just a little bunny."

Vanquished by Vampire Bat

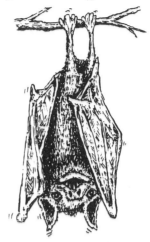

"All I know is that I must soon die, but what I know least is this very death which I cannot escape."
—Pascal, 1670.

Truly marvelous among the adaptations of nature are the changes in forelimbs that allow a mammal to fly, and no other mammal has made this adaptation except the bat. Of the more than 900 species of bats on earth, only three are truly blood-sucking vampires, bats that live entirely off blood: the common vampire, the white-winged vampire and the hairy-legged vampire (*Desmodus, Diaemus* and *Diphylla*). They have no regard for the source of the red fluid. Human to toad, it's just food to the bat. They find suitable habitat primarily in the tropics and subtropics of the Americas.

Vampire bats home in with their keen sense of smell, with remarkable heat receptors in and below their fatty noses and with echolocation (screaming too high pitched for humans to hear and listening for the echo off of whatever they're headed for). With needle-sharp incisors, they bite, preferring in humans a small, blood-filled body part such as finger or toe, nose or cheek. Once they create the characteristic V-shaped wounds, they slobber into the opening, their saliva containing an anticoagulant to keep the blood flowing. Vampire bats don't actually suck, but, instead, lap up the red stuff with their tongues. They'll lap for 20 to 30 minutes if you leave them alone.

One bat would not remove enough blood to kill you. In fact, a half dozen probably wouldn't. To be totally honest, nobody knows exactly how many vampire bats would have to feed for how many minutes before you'd reach your expiration date. Nobody has ever been willing to let them feed that long. The immediate danger is far greater from the germs bats may have in their mouths (see RAVAGED BY RABIES).

Moral: Bats "suck."

Vaporized by Volcano

"Death, the most dreaded of evils, is therefore of no concern to us; for while we exist death is not present, and when death is present we no longer exist."

—Epicurus, Third Century BC.

During every moment of every day about one out of every 10 human earthlings is somewhere where a volcano can get them. Approximately 600 volcanoes are currently labeled "active." Thousands more are "dormant" which means they could go active any second.

Volcanoes are vents or "chimneys" from the enormous reservoir of molten magma inside the earth to the surface of the earth. When gases build up beneath a volcano to the point where something has to give, the molten rock gives because it's softer than the surrounding hard rock. The volcano erupts, and lava flows everywhere, and you may think that lava provides your best chance to die. Not so. Lava actually moves so slow that rare is the human who can't outrun it. But volcanoes have several other ways to make you no longer exist.

(1) Falling ash can bury you, a problem that becomes especially likely if it happens to start raining, since the rain makes the ash heavy.

(2) Pyroclastic flows are horizontally directed blasts from a volcano, blasts that contain ash and small chunks of hot lava, a flood of fire traveling at great speed, a force which vaporizes everything in its path.

(3) Debris (ash and lava fragments) collects near the top of a volcano and, if it gets wet, say from rainfall or snowmelt, it turns into a material similar in consistency to really wet concrete. If the stuff starts to slide, it has been known to travel as far as 60 miles, burying everything in the line of flow.

(4) Volcanic gases, which may slip out even when no eruption is taking place, often contain carbon dioxide and other unbreathable gases which can settle into low-lying spots and choke you to death.

Moral: If you can't take the heat, get out of the kitchen.

Wasted by Walrus

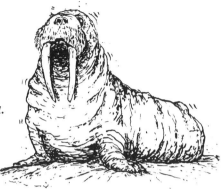

"Do not seek death. Death will find you. But seek the road which makes death a fulfillment."
—Dag Hammarskjold, 1964.

All the pinnipeds of the world (seals, sea lions, walruses) are eaters of flesh, but their diets are limited to fish, squid, octopus, shellfish and occasionally a bird. They have no interest in eating a human, but the largest of the pinnipeds can be dangerous, even life-threatening to humans. Take the walruses, for instance, creatures that mature at nearly a ton-and-a-half for males and a ton for females.

Walruses (*Odobenus rosmarus rosmarus* in the Atlantic, *O. rosmarus divergens* in the Pacific), both sexes, have flattened mollusk-crushing teeth except for their two enormously elongated canines, their tusks. They live only in the northern climes of earth, and they are brightly intelligent with a well-developed fear of humans.

During breeding seasons or when the mothers have young in their keeping, walruses can develop quarrelsome attitudes and have been known to attack passersby and small boats. When wounded, they generally stop at little that holds a promise of retaliation. Walruses will throw their huge bulk at you and, if they land as planned, you will be squashed to a shadow of your former self. Although they don't appear to aim a tusk at you, if a tusk happens to catch you, you'll be ripped from stem to stern. Not exceptionally fast on land, you should be able to outrun an enraged walrus if you have a decent head start.

Moral: A great show of teeth is not necessarily a smile.

Wiped Out by Wart Hog

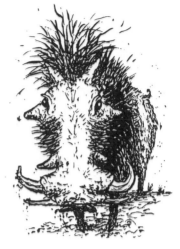

"Death holds no horrors. It is simply the ultimate horror of life."
    –Jean Giraudoux, 1933.

The world enjoys a plethora of wild pigs: javelinas (peccaries) of the southwestern United States, razorbacks of the southeastern United States, wild boars of Europe. Although not given over totally to vegetarianism, they never hunt large animals, such as humans, for food. They do, however, possess short tempers and a determined willingness to kill when aroused. A hunter in Mexico who was chased up a tree once reported: "They were chewing the tree, and climbing over each other trying to get at me. Each shot laid one out, and each shot seemed to make them more and more furious, as they would rush at the tree, and gnaw the bark and wood, while white flakes of froth fell from their mouths."

African swine of the genus *Phacochaerus* are distinguished by large wart-like protuberances on each side of their remarkably fierce faces and by four large, sharp tusks that curve upward from their perpetually sneering lips. Three to four feet long, they are typically reddish-gray in color with a bristly black mane and spinal stripe. They are courageous, ferocious and really dirty fighters. When threatened, or even sometimes just approached, they attack in mass, thrashing wildly from right to left, up and down, with lunges of their powerful necks, wielding their tusks like a mad drunk with a knife in a New York alley. Wart hogs will rip the tendons out of your legs in order to bring you down to their level. But the ripping has only begun. By the time they're satisfied, you'll cover far more square footage than you used to.

Moral: When the pork are out, they may pork out on you.